The Parent Pivot is an innovative and resourceful guide for parents of young adults in emotional distress. With real-world case examples and storytelling, *The Parent Pivot* provides parents with useful coping tools, informational resources, and a new relationship model for responding to the emotional distress of their young adult. More than anything, this marvelous book gives desperate parents some concrete measure of hope.

–**SHERRY CORMIER, PhD,** PSYCHOLOGIST, BEREAVEMENT TRAUMA SPECIALIST, CONSULTANT, AND AUTHOR OF *SWEET SORROW: FINDING ENDURING WHOLENESS AFTER LOSS AND GRIEF*

Reading every chapter, or even every page of this book, powerfully equips a parent (or an aunt, uncle, grandparent, or anyone who loves an emerging adult) with expert knowledge and evidence-based practice, enveloped in thoughtfulness and grace. The authors thoroughly understand the depths and intricacies of being a parent and offer a liberating yet intentional way of living for both the emerging adult and the self.

–**TES TUASON, PhD,** PROFESSOR AND PROGRAM DIRECTOR, CLINICAL MENTAL HEALTH COUNSELING, BROOKS COLLEGE OF HEALTH, UNIVERSITY OF NORTH FLORIDA, JACKSONVILLE

This book serves as an amazing resource for parents whose children are on the cusp of emerging adulthood during these especially challenging times. The authors address concerns of young adults ranging from daily stressors to unhealthy coping behaviors to serious mental health disorders. This book provides help and support in understandable and relatable ways. Most important, this resource equips you with the knowledge and skills necessary to care for yourself as you navigate the demands associated with your evolving role.

–**CLIFF MCKINNEY, PhD,** DEPARTMENT OF PSYCHOLOGY, MISSISSIPPI STATE UNIVERSITY

This book is an exceptionally valuable resource for parents and caretakers who are trying to help their young adult children cope with emotional distress and more serious mental health disorders. The authors very clearly describe the challenges that can emerge during this critical developmental period and offer practical suggestions for how best to support their children. The authors have many years of experience and their expertise contributes to the credibility of the content of the book. The real-life case studies, the conversational writing style, and the focus of hope in the last chapter should appeal to parents who are struggling to help their children navigate a difficult period in their development.

–ANN VERNON, PhD, PROFESSOR EMERITA, UNIVERSITY OF
NORTHERN IOWA, CEDAR FALLS

THE
PARENT
PIVOT

WHAT TO DO WHEN YOUR YOUNG ADULT
IS IN PSYCHOLOGICAL DISTRESS

THE

PARENT

PIVOT

LYNNE CARROLL, PhD, ABPP

PAULA J. GILROY, EdD

MIKAL CRAWFORD, EdD

 AMERICAN PSYCHOLOGICAL ASSOCIATION

Published by
American Psychological Association
750 First Street, NE
Washington, DC 20002
https://www.apa.org

Order Department
https://www.apa.org/pubs/books
order@apa.org

Typeset in Sabon by Circle Graphics, Inc., Reisterstown, MD

Printer: Sheridan Books, Chelsea, MI
Cover Designer: Mark Karis

"Spectacles" icon by Shiva, from thenounproject.com CC BY 3.0
"Lightening Bolt" icon by Muneer A.Safiah, from thenounproject.com CC BY 3.0
"tote bag" icon by iconixar, from thenounproject.com CC BY 3.0

Library of Congress Cataloging-in-Publication Data

Names: Carroll, Lynne, author. | Gilroy, Paula J., author. | Crawford, Mikal C., author.
Title: The parent pivot : what to do when your young adult is in psychological distress / by Lynne Carroll, Paula J. Gilroy, and Mikal Crawford.
Description: Washington, DC : American Psychological Association, [2025] | Includes bibliographical references and index. | Audience term: Parents
Identifiers: LCCN 2024045365 (print) | LCCN 2024045366 (ebook) | ISBN 9781433843631 (paperback) | ISBN 9781433843648 (ebook)
Subjects: LCSH: Young adults—Psychology. | Young adults—Mental health. | Crisis intervention (Mental health services)
Classification: LCC RC451.4.Y67 C37 2025 (print) | LCC RC451.4.Y67 (ebook) | DDC 616.8900835—dc23/eng/20250205
LC record available at https://lccn.loc.gov/2024045365
LC ebook record available at https://lccn.loc.gov/2024045366

https://doi.org/10.1037/0000459-000

Printed in the United States of America

10 9 8 7 6 5 4 3 2 1

This book is for parents of young adults everywhere.
We lovingly dedicate it to the Butterfly
who has inspired our journey.

CONTENTS

ACKNOWLEDGMENTS

We would like to express our profound gratitude to the many young adults and parents whose stories inspired us to write this book. For all those clients we helped along the way, and those we might not have reached, we feel privileged to have learned from you. The personal stories you shared provided us with the motivation and fueled the perseverance we needed to stay the course over the lengthy process of writing this book. The cases we follow throughout the book are based on a number of client stories we have heard over the years. Salient features have been changed to protect the identity and maintain confidentiality of our former clients and their families.

We thank Drs. Tes Tuason, Sherry Cormier, and Ann Vernon, whose professional insights were invaluable. We are deeply appreciative to various early readers including Gail Kelley, Louise Odle, Jan Kellner, Barbara Palmiter, Sharon Wilson-Barker, Dr. John Yasenchak, Dr. Deb Drew, Mary Farrell, Paula Titon, and Sharon Matthews, who provided helpful feedback and perspective on our journey with this book.

We are grateful to the American Psychological Association team, especially Stevie Davall, Beth Hatch, Elizabeth Budd, and Elizabeth Brace, for their belief in our project and their guidance in seeing it across the finish line. Thank you to Jason Wells who spearheaded the marketing of our book.

We are grateful to the many family members and friends who supported us throughout the writing process. Our families were patient, understanding, and nurturing beyond measure. We offer special thanks to: Debbie Price (Lynne), Phil Patton, Elise Patton, Christine Gilroy (Paula), John Lowe, Katie McLaughlin, and Erin McLaughlin (Mikal).

It is important to recognize the collaborative nature of writing this book and the challenges inherent in three different perspectives, three different geographical locations, and three very strong and, at times, differing opinions! Over the course of the last three years, through the COVID-19 pandemic and its aftermath, we connected on Zoom calls, sometimes two or three times a week, for marathon sessions as we moved this project from an idea to a completed work.

THE
PARENT
PIVOT

THE PIVOTING WHEEL

In a world rife with tension, disagreement, and chaos of many kinds, there is one thing most people will agree on: We want the best for our children. Many also come to realize that our parenting job doesn't end when our children become legal adults at age 18. Indeed, for many of us, our journeys become more complicated as our children strive to make their own way in the adult world. Most likely you were a hands-on parent for 17 years, and as such you exercised control over many of the decisions in your child's life and the choices they made. Now, however, they may legally take up the reins of their lives, making important decisions and leaving you on the sidelines. The adult world they are entering is complex and uncertain, full of possibilities and pitfalls. Likewise, as parents you are moving into uncharted waters yourselves. Psychologists have viewed the period between ages 18 and 29 to be a distinct stage of development characterized by multiple transitions. Individuals in this age group—whom we refer to interchangeably as *young adults*, *emerging adults*, and *adult children*—often undergo some form of psychological distress. Parents, whose lives are intertwined with their children's, also experience their own stress as their young adults are given the green light to govern their own lives.

This book is for parents whose emerging adults are experiencing some form of psychological or emotional distress; this can range from

3

mild symptoms to more serious mental health disorders (e.g., generalized anxiety disorder, major depressive disorder, bipolar disorder). Our book provides you with much needed information to assist you in understanding your adult child's symptoms and in navigating our current mental health system. Additionally, we address unhealthy behaviors (e.g., substance misuse, internet misuse, unhealthy eating and exercise) and high-risk behaviors (e.g., self-injury) that young adults may use to manage their distress. These maladaptive coping strategies create distress and fear in the parents and complicate their relationships and communications with their emerging adults.

As psychologists, the three of us have more than a century of combined professional work with young adults in clinical and educational settings as well as experience working with parents and other adults on wellness and well-being. We offer you our collective knowledge and experience to help you maintain your sanity while you grapple with the challenges and changes in your parenting role. We strongly believe that lifelong learning empowers each and every one of us. In addition, two of us have direct experience parenting young adults. Each of us has experienced, personally and professionally, the struggles young adults go through as they make decisions and move forward with their lives. We have also confronted the more serious challenges of young adults with mental illnesses that derailed their plans and threatened to stop their forward progress completely. In addition, we have encountered the tragic circumstances of young adults who make serious self-injurious gestures or die by suicide. The devastating impact on parents, other family members, and friends is very real. Such losses also take a toll on the mental health professionals who are either directly or indirectly involved. We are writing this book in the hope of assisting parents to find the help they need to support their young adults across a variety of circumstances, while not losing sight of their own needs or compromising their own well-being.

THE PIVOTING WHEEL FOR PARENTS

Pivoting is the ability to shift course and move in a new direction as the situation demands. By the time you become the parent of a young adult, you have adapted or pivoted many times to suit the developmental phases and life circumstances of your child. From the day you brought your infant or child into your home you realized that your regular routine was no longer viable. You made the pivot to caretaker when you started to put the needs of your child center stage and move your own needs to the side. Sleep was one of the first disruptions in normal routine, and there were many others. As this little person began to grow and move around in the world, you continued to adapt to accommodate their ever-changing developmental needs. You learned the importance of communicating effectively, establishing boundaries, and setting rules and enforcing them with consistency. You also learned how and when to be flexible to accommodate the changing circumstances and needs of your child. As they grew, you likely gave your child increasing freedom and relaxed the need to control their every move. Some of the decisions you made during this time were relatively easy, while others were difficult and no doubt caused considerable stress for you. You learned how the demands associated with parenting quite often necessitate that you attend to your own self-care. If you are like many parents, however, you may have put taking care of yourself at the bottom of your to-do list.

As you will see, pivoting is about adapting to the situation rather than rigidly adhering to old patterns of behavior which are typically not effective in new circumstances. This process is fundamental to the work of a parent. By the time your child becomes a mature adult, you may make as many as four pivots in your parenting journey to accommodate developmental phases and life circumstances. It might help to envision a well-greased axle on a big wheel that allows you to turn readily to meet new demands for yourself and your young adult (see Figure 1).

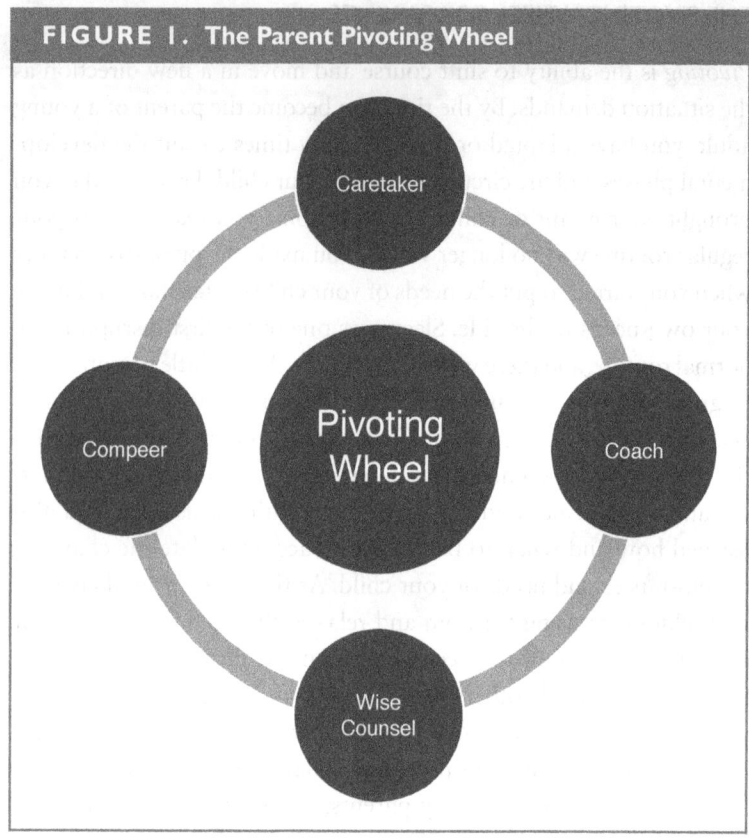

FIGURE 1. The Parent Pivoting Wheel

As your child enters the stage of emerging adulthood, you may be ready to make a pivot from the *caretaker* role where you have been handling the physical and emotional needs of your young child to becoming a *coach* as your young adult heads out into the world. You pull back from hands-on caretaking and enter a new role of guiding and teaching your young adult as they mature and grow. You are no longer "doing for" but rather modeling effective behavior and actively guiding your adult child. *Wise counsel* is the third pivot point in which you are more like an on-call consultant in your adult child's life. A wise counsel is available when their adult child approaches them for advice but emphasizes that the final choice rests with the young adult. The challenge for the wise counsel is to adopt a supportive and nonjudgmental tone and to respond to your young adult when asked for an opinion or advice. A wise counsel does not jump in and fix the problem. During the latter part of the emerging adult stage, it may be possible for parents to make yet a fourth pivot to that of *compeer* in which we enter a role as an equal with our offspring. Think of this as a combination of "companion" and "peer." Our use of the word companion is intended to mean a relationship of equals who enjoy each other's company, sometimes without having to say a word. We explain these pivots in greater detail in the coming chapters.

WHEN DO I PIVOT?

As the parent of a young adult, you can determine the appropriate role for a given situation based on two factors: first and foremost is their level of functioning, and second is their level of distress. It is important to understand that your young adult may function fairly well even in the face of considerable distress. There isn't a simple formula here for knowing when to pivot. Please keep this in mind as we continue.

Generally speaking, functioning declines as distress rises. You may intuitively move toward the more hands-on role of a caretaker in this situation. On the flip side, usually the higher the young adult's functioning, the lower the level of distress. In this instance your instincts may tell you to back off and adopt the wise counsel or compeer role.

Things get tricky, though, when functioning and distress don't neatly line up. For example, even when your young adult is functioning moderately well, they may still be experiencing considerable psychological distress. However, they might be able to hear what you have to say and make effective decisions. Conversely, your young adult could be functioning poorly with a relatively low level of distress.

Let's consider the decision of when to pivot by using a continuum as a tool. In Figure 2, you see a 10-point continuum that depicts a range of functioning from minimal to high. Based on Steinberg's (2023) work, at the high end of functioning known as *flourishing*, the young adult exhibits the following: a strong sense of engagement in daily life; strong connections with others; optimism and hope for the future; strong motivation and interest in work, academics, and hobbies; *grit* (i.e., perseverance when things get tough), and a sense of joy. At the lower end of this continuum, we see emerging adults who lack these same qualities; according to Steinberg, they are *floundering*.

Just as we offer a continuum for level of functioning, we offer a continuum as a tool to help you think about where your young adult may fall in terms of their psychological distress. In Figure 3, you see a 10-point continuum that depicts a range of distress from minimal to severe. Based on Kessler et al.'s (2002) work on the assessment of

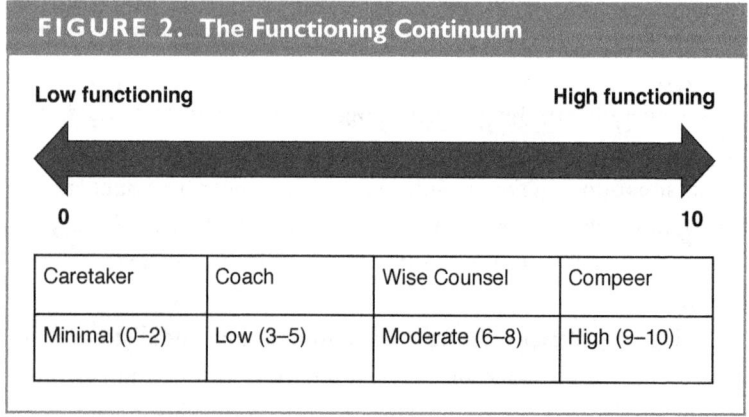

FIGURE 2. The Functioning Continuum

Low functioning   High functioning

0   10

Caretaker	Coach	Wise Counsel	Compeer
Minimal (0–2)	Low (3–5)	Moderate (6–8)	High (9–10)

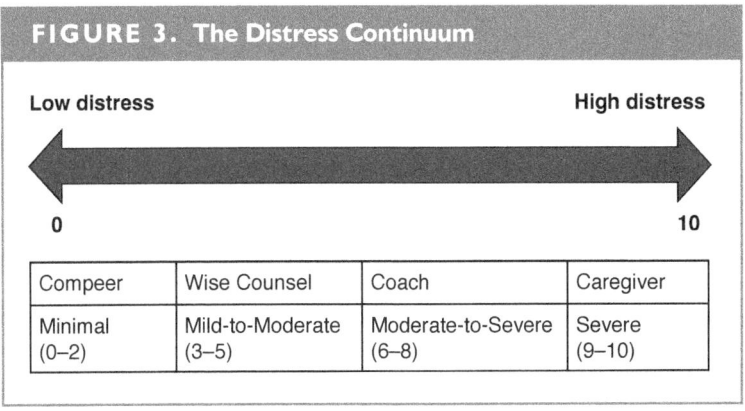

FIGURE 3. The Distress Continuum

Low distress   **High distress**

0   10

Compeer	Wise Counsel	Coach	Caregiver
Minimal (0–2)	Mild-to-Moderate (3–5)	Moderate-to-Severe (6–8)	Severe (9–10)

psychological distress, at the severe end of our continuum, the young adult experiences excessive nervousness, restlessness or fidgeting, extreme tiredness, severe depression, hopelessness, and worthlessness. In such situations, the ability to think clearly and rationally is severely hampered by the distress, and your young adult is not able to hear what you have to say. In addition, their ability to function effectively at work or school is impaired. At the minimal end of the continuum, your young adult has little to none of these signs of distress. In such circumstances, they are handling their daily lives effectively and are likely able to engage in healthy interactions with you. They are also more receptive to new ideas.

Knowing when to pivot is not easy. There is no simple recipe or formula to follow. Instead, this process requires you to use your understanding of your adult child and the knowledge you will gain from this book to make an informed assessment of what your young adult needs at this particular stage in their life. It is also important to note that the process of pivoting is not a linear one. At any time, you can pivot to a previous point given the needs of the situation. Even as you pivot to wise counsel or compeer, caretaker and coach are viable pivots when necessary.

Imagine, for example, that your emerging adult develops a serious physical illness such as cancer. You are likely to pivot to caretaker initially until you have enough information and clarity to decide what to do next. You will also need the coach and wise counsel skills to help you. Remaining in caretaker mode can actually be detrimental to you and your adult child in such a situation. Obviously, decisions about when and which role to pivot to are not easy. A mental health issue is no different, and your ability to make necessary pivots is crucial—not only for your young adult but also for your own well-being. Regardless of which pivot you make in any given situation, respect and support of your young adult's autonomy and independence are essential.

When you make any of these pivots, you carry the skills from the previous roles with you; each skill builds on the previous ones. Developing these skills takes time, as parents need to master foundational skills first before moving on to more complex ones. This is quite similar to the way we learned mathematics in school. Remember early on how you were asked to recognize numbers and over time learned how to add and subtract, and then progressed on to learn more complex operations like multiplication and division? Algebra and geometry followed after the basics were mastered.

The needs of your young adult certainly impact your decisions regarding the pivots. But what about you, the parent? How might you influence what role you should play for a given situation? What if you are suffering significant distress watching your adult child suffer, and thus believe you need to step in and fix things? Psychological flexibility is necessary when your adult child is in emotional distress. You will need to develop the capacity to pivot to and from your parenting roles to engage in specific behaviors that may not be in your repertoire, while simultaneously self-regulating your own distress. We view your level of distress as more an indication of how much you need self-care, rather than what role is most beneficial to your adult child right now. Self-care is always important, but it becomes even more important when you are struggling because of your adult child's emotional pain. Developing this self-awareness is crucial because addressing your own distress is vital to the pivoting process. The techniques we share for self-care will help you. Remember, taking care of yourself is vital, however, self-care is not something that most parents are inclined to do.

In the chapters that follow, we provide you with further information about your parenting roles and guide you through these pivot points. We offer tools for making your journey more doable. And most importantly, we discuss the challenges many parents face when their emerging adults exhibit signs of psychological distress, including more serious mental illnesses. As you pivot to meet oncoming changes and demands in both your life and that of your emerging adult, you improve your mental and physical well-being as well as overall resilience. Resilience, or the ability to adapt to changing situations, can be a powerful ally in your journey as a parent and a person.

TWO COMMON THEMES

One theme you will notice throughout the book, which we have already introduced in the previous section, is the importance of taking care of yourself while you respond to the challenges of having a distressed emerging adult. That well-worn cliche of putting your own oxygen mask on first before turning to help your seatmate is essential to keep in mind. If you can't function, you will be of no use to your adult child. To that end, we also offer skills for handling your own stress and managing your well-being. Our overall physical, mental, and emotional well-being is often severely taxed, and stress levels may be off the charts at times as we continue to adapt our parenting to meet the needs of our adult children. This is especially true when our emerging adults show signs of something more than just growing pains, and we as parents question whether there is something more serious happening with them. Our worry meter kicks into high gear and our well-being likely plummets while we navigate the complexities and challenges of parenting our adult children.

The second theme you will notice, which we also introduced in the previous section, is the use of a continuum approach throughout the book. We view behaviors and mental health issues not as either–or distinct categories, but rather in terms of degrees of health or functionality. This applies to your young adult's behavior as well as your own. We live in a world that likes to box things into neat categories such as good versus bad or yes versus no. Such categories suggest there is a clear judgment in one direction or the other. Experience teaches us, however, that the lines between such distinctions are far from clear. Life is not black or white, and many of us are uncomfortable living in the "gray" area. We want clear, definitive answers, and such answers don't often exist. Even in the mental health field, the professional guidelines outlined in the *Diagnostic and Statistical Manual of Mental Disorders* (American Psychiatric Association, 2022) now apply this continuum approach in diagnosing mental health disorders. In other words, the focus is on the degree to which a person is impaired by their symptoms rather than the presence or absence of these symptoms.

We all encounter stress in our lives, and it often varies in intensity. On any given day, your stress may start out as minimal. As the day continues, and you are stuck in traffic and late for an appointment, it will likely rise. Once you are exiting the appointment and heading to lunch with a friend, it may subside a bit. It is fluid and not stuck in an on-versus-off mode. So, too, might your young adult's behaviors fall on a continuum of functionality. Sleeping in on any given day is not uncommon for young adults, and few parents would bat an eye at that. However, sleeping in for 4 or 5 days in a row and missing work or classes may raise your level of concern.

To the question of "When should I worry?" we say there are no quick, easy, or definitive answers; each young adult and their circumstances are unique. However, we offer information to guide you in recognizing warning signs and red flags that indicate your young adult may be sliding down a slippery slope. We believe that behaviors, such as those resulting in impairment in daily living tasks (work, school, personal self-care), are the clearest markers of potential problems. The key is to catch the behaviors before they spiral into a more serious situation. The earlier the intervention, the better the prognosis and overall quality of life for parents, young adults, and family.

SPECTACLES, LIGHTNING BOLTS, AND TOTE BAGS

 Throughout the book, we present up-to-date information to empower you by helping you better understand what is going on with yourself as well as your young adult. Like the turtle who pulls his head into the shell when frightened, we sometimes also pull back in the face of new and unsettling information. We encourage you to lean into the discomfort you might feel and not shy away from what you might discover. Watch for the symbol of a pair of spectacles as a signpost for potentially complex material that may require a closer reading to fully understand.

It is likely you will experience discomfort with some of the material you read in this book. Just as we tell clients in their first session, therapy can involve uncovering deeper and sometimes unexpected and intense emotions. This is often unsettling, particularly early on in the therapy process. However, counseling can offer the chance to learn more effective strategies to manage your feelings while also gaining a new perspective on your situation. Likewise, you as a parent are apt to feel some distress as you work your way through the book. This is part of the process of learning new information and gaining a deeper understanding of your young adult and their psychological distress. In addition, you may also be realizing some things about your own behavior, past and present, that could be upsetting for you. We offer calming techniques along the way to help you as you continue your journey through the book. We encourage you to have compassion for yourself as you continue through the book and make use of the calming techniques offered in the chapters. Like the lightning bolt in a thunderstorm, we can't predict when the jolt will hit you, however, we place a lightning bolt where we think a jolt is likely to occur.

 Throughout the book, we help you fill up a metaphorical tote bag with tools to take with you on your journey as you move forward with your young adult. In our respective clinical work, each of us quickly discovered that although therapy takes time, our clients often wanted and needed a "to-go" bag at the end of each session, something tangible to take home. Therefore, each chapter includes several tools because we know that no single tool is sufficient to get any job done. You will see this symbol throughout the book to indicate the tools you can put in your tote bag as you move along.

Most artisans practice their craft by finding the right personal "fit" in terms of tools and working hard. Please note that while the tools we offer you are supported by research, some will be a better fit for you than others. We encourage you to read through all the tools; in time you will figure out which will work best for you.

INTRODUCING OUR CASES

The power of stories has long been understood by people around the world. The field of neuroscience (study of the brain) with the use of brain imaging now adds scientific proof to the idea that stories have the power to both inform and transform us in profound ways. Brain scans of the storyteller and the listener show that their brains mirror one another. Areas of the listener's brain that control perspective-taking are activated, something that does not happen when the individual is simply listening to a lecture of facts or statistics (Chang et al., 2024; Stephens et al., 2010).

As clinicians and teachers, we also deeply appreciate the power of stories and narrative in our work with clients and students. To engage you, our readers, more fully, we use the stories of four families throughout our book. We draw on our work with clients and incorporate their stories, all the while knowing these stories do not fully reflect the range of human experiences that exist in the world today. We have changed certain details in these narratives to protect the identities and to maintain the confidentiality of our clients and their family members. As you move from one chapter to the next, you will take the journey with our parents—Claire and Stan, Lucia and Arturo, Rachel, and Pete. You will temporarily inhabit their worlds offer a bird's-eye view of the many challenges that await our parents as their emerging adults experience mental health issues. Although we appreciate the vast diversity and complexity that exist in today's families, we hope you may find yourself identifying with aspects of our parents' experiences.

While some young adults launch successfully, others start off well initially and then fall backward. There is a third group that never gets off the ground. We want to introduce you to four young adults from different backgrounds who appear to be launching successfully. As you read the introduction by their mother or father, do you notice any signs, subtle or otherwise, that a storm could be brewing? As parents, we don't want to notice such signs, however, it is important to understand that what you may see initially is not necessarily an accurate reflection of the young adult's overall well-being or their progress toward adulthood. Let's listen as each parent introduces their adult child.

Anne's mother, Claire, said the following:

Stan and I celebrated Anne's graduation from high school because it meant a new beginning for her, and she was excited to move on with her life as a college freshman. Both of us were supportive of Anne's choice of history as a major, given her love of ancient history. At the same time, Anne and I had many conversations about possible career goals for history majors. I believed it was important for Anne to be aware of some future career options for whatever major she chose. I also talked with her about the importance of requesting academic accommodations or assistance for a learning disability, which was diagnosed in third grade. However, Anne refused to request help. I can't say I was surprised as Anne always struggled to accept the diagnosis of dyslexia, but I very much wanted her to have a solid academic support system in place. At first, college offered a very positive change for Anne. She lived on campus in a residence hall and cultivated friendships quickly. Her grades were good, and she kept her job at the local grocery store. Anne appeared content and happy during her first semester, and I felt relieved.

Daniel's father, Arturo, said the following:

What can I say about my son, Daniel? My family is from Guatemala. My father, Daniel's grandfather, emigrated here, and he and my mother settled in a part of town that is mostly Hispanic. It was a rough place to grow up. Lots of the kids who grew up around me turned out to be *pandillero* (gang members). My father was a no-nonsense, stern man, and he beat into me that I had to work hard. He helped me make a good connection so I got myself a job as an assembly-line worker at the auto plant, and I worked my way up from the bottom to line supervisor.

I met Lucia, and we got married and had our two kids when we were pretty young. I made up my mind that my son would go to college; no son of mine was going to have to struggle growing up the way I did. Daniel was such a good kid. He's always loved baseball. On his Little League team, he had to be better than everyone on the team because I was the coach back then. He didn't want anyone on his team to think he had an edge with me being his coach and all. In high school, he was a "cleanup hitter" on the team, and I went to as many of Daniel's home games as I could—even switched my schedule around so that I could work nights. Daniel's *amá* and I are proud of how hard he's worked to overcome his ADHD to get into college. He wants to go pro but I told him he's got to have a career to fall back on just in case.

Jessie's mom, Rachel, said the following:

Jessie is a great kid. She had to grow up pretty quickly after her father was killed in Afghanistan. As my older child, she helped with her younger brother and took on a lot of responsibility at home. I work as an EMT and am called out for emergencies at odd hours, so she covered for me a lot. I really wanted her to go on to college after high school, but Jessie has always been self-directed, and she chose to work full time instead. She's been on her own for several years and has done very well. She's a manager now at Planet Fitness, and I am so proud of her. I guess not everyone has to go to college.

Ian's father, Pete, said the following:

As a single father with an adopted biracial son, I have walked a tightrope sometimes trying to make sure that Ian gets all the love and support he needs while trying not to "father hen" him. I am very proud of Ian, he graduated with high honors from high school and has completed his first year of college. He has always been a bit reserved, preferring to go his own way. Yet he had a great group of friends in high school, and I would say he was a popular kid. In my work as a high school physics teacher, I have seen a lot of young people take wrong turns and end up in trouble with the law or injured in some way. Ian bypassed the nastiness of that and worked hard to achieve the scholarships that helped him through his first year.

Clearly, these parents are proud of their young adults, and optimistic for their futures. They have all successfully graduated from high school and have plans for what they want to do. Anne, Daniel, and Ian are attending college, and Jessie has launched herself on a different path where she lives on her own and has responsible employment in a managerial position. For Claire, Stan, Arturo, Lucia, Rachel, and Pete, their parenting work has paid off, and they can begin to relax their efforts with their young adult. They may begin to dream of the possibility in the future of a friendship with their adult child. Such a new relationship might involve spending time together without an agenda or expectations. We continue to follow these parents and their young adults as we turn our attention to the process of pivoting.

HOW THE BOOK IS ORGANIZED

Our book is organized into three parts, with each section building on the previous one. If you've picked up this book, you might identify with the feelings of frustration, anger, fear, disappointment, among others, often expressed by parents of adult children who are struggling with the adulting process. Part I, "OMG! I Thought I Was Done," captures this sentiment. In these chapters, we discuss various factors that contribute to some of the commonly observed changes that occur in young people during the emerging adulthood stage. We offer our parenting model, which we call the "pivoting wheel" to help you conceptualize your various roles as a parent. The wheel is a tool to help you better appreciate and understand the fluid nature of parenting at this stage, especially in situations when your young adult is experiencing psychological distress. Our aim is to help you in thinking about when and how you might pivot to a role that best addresses the changing demands and circumstances you and your young adult may face.

Part II, "Upside Down and Inside Out," refers to the upheaval you will likely experience when your adult child is in psychological distress. We aid you in better understanding the continuum of distress ranging from mild anxiety and depression to more serious mental health disorders. Here we empower you with information and skills necessary to engage effectively in difficult dialogues with your adult child. We also assist you in better understanding the complex process of getting a diagnosis if there is a mental illness and the sometimes nightmarish challenge of finding and getting into effective treatment. We provide you with practical advice to use in the selection of mental health care providers and evidence-based treatment approaches. We offer useful tips on how to respond if your adult child shuts you out of the process. We provide tools both for understanding and coping with feelings of loss that can be so overwhelming for parents.

Part III, "Right Side Up Again," refers to the ability to shift from focusing on the needs of your distressed young adult to addressing your own self-care. When you are "right side up," you are better able to achieve a healthy balance between caring for yourself and others, including your young adult. The linchpin of self-care is a combination of building resilience and practicing self-compassion.

We conclude each chapter with "Points to Pocket," a list of key takeaways we want you to grasp as you read the chapter. We are with you every step of the way with tools and assistance to help you deal with what you are feeling and manage the stress this experience can generate. As you learn to engage in compassion for yourself, you will be in a better position to help your young adult navigate their own troubled waters.

We strongly recommend that you read each chapter in order, as each chapter builds on the previous ones. Remember the symbols of the tote bag, lightning bolt, and spectacles as signposts along the way.

Are you ready? Pick up that tote bag and let's begin.

I

OMG! I THOUGHT I WAS DONE

CHAPTER 1

A WORLD IN CHAOS

Adulthood is like the vet, and we're all the dogs that were
excited for the car ride until we realized where we're going.
— Anita Room

Feeling unsettled? Confused? A bit anxious, perhaps? You're not alone! We live and parent today in a very chaotic world which often makes little or no sense. The sheer number of challenges we face, from the COVID-19 pandemic to natural disasters such as hurricanes, tornadoes, and wildfires, to unsettling legal assaults on rights formerly guaranteed by law, to turbulent and divisive political rhetoric, all these play havoc with our sense of order in the world and common civility in our interactions with each other. We have news streaming 24/7 and the latest hurricane devastation videos or political hype giddily dished up by the cable news pundits eager to grab headlines and viewers. For many of us, the turmoil in the world today, mudslides, flooding, and multiple mass fatality shootings every week, make it difficult to let go of the need to protect our children regardless of their age. It seems that danger is lurking everywhere, from schools to movie theaters, medical facilities to public transportation, and even the local mall. Where is the safe haven we need in our communities? If nowhere is safe, parent anxiety and stress hit a new high and make it difficult to engage in nonemotional thinking and behavior. Being able to calm oneself and regulate reactions is crucial to being adequately prepared for the demands of these difficult times.

Navigating this chaos becomes doubly challenging when you are also navigating the new world of parenting your adult child. To borrow a term from the organizational management field (Bennett & Lemoine, 2014), we live in a "VUCA" environment (volatile, uncertain, complex, and ambiguous) that tests our ability to function effectively.

In this chapter, we offer you a picture of the young adult population against the backdrop of our current social, cultural, legal, and political climate and provide a picture of the new and more complex process of becoming an adult. We describe how this VUCA environment impacts the emerging adult experience. Parenting at any time requires the ability to pivot, meaning to change direction to meet the needs of the current situation. In this chapter and throughout the book, we offer a model of pivoting that is especially germane to parenting during emerging adulthood. In our opinion, pivoting is rendered that much more difficult because of the VUCA environment. We describe the process of pivoting to keep yourself centered as you parent your young adult.

ADULTHOOD IN A NEW LIGHT

Think back to your own journey to adulthood. Traditionally, being an adult meant finishing your education, getting a job, leaving home, getting married, and having children. Adulthood was a destination, a distinct point along the developmental continuum. You jumped the hoops, landed on your feet, and arrived at the destination of full-fledged adulthood. More recently, however, young people are finding that economic and social changes have extended schooling, delayed the attainment of meaningful work, and led to postponement of marriage and childbearing. At present, there doesn't seem to be a uniform set of criteria that defines adulthood. Additionally, there appears to be much more of a process involved in becoming an adult, rather than a clear arrival point. Today's young adults unfortunately seem to struggle with the idea of process because they are so focused on the outcome. Most of us are left to ponder, what does "being an adult" really mean?

Regardless of whether your young adult enrolls in higher education, they are beginning to make important decisions that will affect their future. As they struggle with these new life tasks, you begin your transition as a parent. In Chapter 2, we say more about your transition.

You and your emerging adult are engaged in a parallel process in which you both struggle to redefine yourselves. By this we mean that each of you is experiencing your own developmental transition as you continue your journeys together. As you both grapple with the shifting dynamics of new roles, you must also contend with the stress of living in a volatile and chaotic world.

SO, WHAT IS THIS EMERGING ADULTHOOD?

Psychologist Jeffrey Arnett (2000, 2007) first introduced the term *emerging adulthood* to describe a population of young people who are experiencing a prolonged journey toward adulthood. Arnett sees emerging adulthood as a distinct developmental stage, not an extension of adolescence or a preadult phase, and the tasks associated with this stage of adulting must be viewed through a different lens. According to Arnett, becoming an adult is a complex and lengthy process that involves exploration of one's identity, relationships, career interests, and the development of a sense of meaning and purpose in one's life. Perhaps no other stage, besides infancy, involves such dynamic and complex changes on so many levels (e.g., emotional, social; Wood et al., 2018). Even the brains of emerging adults are still developing, especially in the prefrontal cortex, the area associated with planning, problem-solving, and control of impulses. When it comes to making decisions, mature adult brains are better wired to manage impulsivity and less influenced by emotions, rewards, and social acceptance.

Emerging adulthood involves instability and self-focus. It is also a hopeful time characterized by optimism about the possibilities that exist for oneself. For Arnett and his colleagues, the markers for adulthood are not defined solely by events such as moving out of the home, finding a job, marrying/partnering, and so on. Instead, adulthood means accepting responsibility for oneself, making independent decisions, and becoming financially self-reliant. In our own experiences with young adults and through our research, we found this population to be a kaleidoscope of characteristics. They are diverse (Settersten et al., 2015), and their individual experiences are far from universal. In general, emerging adults experience more prolonged educational pathways and associated debts, rising housing costs, and rising median ages of marriage and parenthood.

A helpful way to think about your emerging adult is by using Laurence Steinberg's (2023) description of *flourishing and floundering*. Steinberg has studied adolescent and emerging adulthood stages of development, most recently how today's young adults are faring in their journeys toward adulthood. In combination, these qualities indicate where the young adult is on the continuum between flourishing and floundering. Throughout this book, we use Steinberg's definition of flourishing when referring to young adults who are high functioning and apply our continuum approach to capture the level at which a young adult is functioning.

Floundering, at the opposite end of the functioning continuum, describes stalled emerging adults who tend to remain dependent, financially and otherwise, on their parents. They struggle to find and maintain a job or to commit to completing a college degree;

they tend to start and quit jobs, activities, or educational programs when they feel overwhelmed or unhappy, as if they are purposely avoiding responsibility.

ARE TODAY'S EMERGING ADULTS FLOUNDERING?

Both popular media and professional journals have described many young adults, but certainly not all, as floundering, stalled, and failures to launch (McConville, 2020). Although it is not known what percentage of young adults might be "floundering," one national survey documented 63% of parents reported some level of fear that their emerging adult would not become a full-fledged adult (Lowe & Arnett, 2020). Some, but not all, young adults engage in unhealthy substance use and other problematic behaviors such as unhealthy eating, lack of exercise and sedentary lifestyles, and internet misuse. They appear unmotivated and disinterested in interacting socially. They also report feeling anxious about falling behind their peers in meeting the markers for becoming an adult. Many emerging adults are described as indecisive, overwhelmed, ambivalent, and lacking resilience (Guare et al., 2019; Konstam, 2013; McConville, 2020).

In both popular media and research, emerging adults are frequently depicted as lacking in basic life skills and self-discipline. Certainly, some young adults make commitments to jobs, social engagements, academic tasks, and other obligations and then don't follow through. Others struggle with organization and forget appointments, misplace their backpacks, or lose their keys. McConville (2020) used the term *administrative responsibility* to describe such basic life tasks as meeting deadlines, keeping appointments, paying bills, and changing the oil in the car. For young adults, administrative responsibility, otherwise known as executive skills, translates into the ability to manage essential details of daily living including being able to handle finances, car insurance and repairs, schedule medical appointments, locate apartments, and understand and sign leases. Some of the difficulties associated with administrative responsibility may be a byproduct of the sheer number of life tasks and an overwhelming number of choices. Schwartz's (2004) analysis of "tyranny of choices" (p. 70) fits nicely here. For emerging adults, having too many possibilities creates anxiety and the fear that one will mistakenly choose the "wrong" option. Alternatively, as we explore later in Chapter 2, young adults' deficiencies in self-management tasks could also be the result of parents overcompensating and doing too much for their children throughout their lives.

Ultimately, there are many reasons why your young adult may have deficiencies in administrative responsibility and why some parents seem to overfunction. Later in this chapter, we explore in greater detail some other factors or "stones in the road" that contribute to these behaviors. Keep in mind the continuum, and understand that there are degrees of flourishing and floundering; it is not an all-or-nothing distinction.

Today's emerging adults experience positives such as mutually closer relationships with parents compared with earlier generations. They may often spend more time with their parents and engage in healthy, mature adult conversations, resulting in parents and their adult children remaining more connected. Of course, although some young adults have stronger connections and close relationships with their parents, this is not always the case, even if they live in close proximity to their parents or in their parents' home. To establish their own autonomy, emerging adults can also exhibit ambivalent behaviors toward their parents, waffling back and forth between seeking closeness and emotionally distancing themselves (Steinberg, 2023). Young adults may be open and overly talkative one day and distant and aloof the next. These behaviors can be confusing and frustrating for parents. At times, parents may feel disappointed, as though they are more invested in the relationship than their adult child—a feeling that can often leave them with a sense of vulnerability.

Many emerging adults have a sense of optimism about themselves and their personal futures, although not necessarily about the world they are inheriting. However, socioeconomic and societal trends may temper such personal optimism. Their exploration of career paths and job opportunities at this point in their lives is an important part of the "adulting" process, but it may be limited by socioeconomic factors largely out of their control. Socioeconomic trends influence one's striving for independence and autonomy.

Obviously, the concerns for parents of some young adults are warranted. Experts agree that emerging adults are anxious, probably even more so now than in previous generations (Arnett et al., 2014; Lythcott-Haims, 2021; McConville, 2020). This increase in anxiety may be due to the many new challenges facing today's emerging adults. We refer to these challenges as stones in the road.

STONES IN THE ROAD

The road to adulthood has always been tricky for many young people. In the current unsettled environment, the hurdles are even more formidable than for past generations. We turn our attention now to some of the significant "stones," or factors that may impinge on your adult child's journey toward adulthood.

Socioeconomic and Cultural Issues

Changes in our economy over the past 20 years have dictated that young adults need financial assistance from their parents, regardless of social class. Although polls vary slightly, at present more than half of parents of young adults provide financial support to their adult children with the most common support in the form of household expenses such as groceries, rent, and utilities; cell phone bills; and streaming subscriptions (Pew Research Center, 2024). At times, this period of extended financial support of emerging adults can be a source of strain between parents and their adult children. Experts agree the single most vexing and contentious area of conflict between parents and young adults is probably finances (Lowe & Arnett, 2020).

Recent sociocultural events such as gun violence, mass shootings, and other forms of victimization make a parent's job of protecting and providing for their children more difficult. Because so many mass shootings have occurred in public schools, homeschooling is more attractive than it used to be when we considered children's safety in school a "given." Likewise, shootings on college campuses have increased significantly in recent decades leaving both young adults and their parents with significant safety concerns. Such shootings have resulted in traumatization for all involved, directly or indirectly.

Discrimination

Systemic racism and other forms of discrimination associated with sex, ethnicity, nationality, immigrant status, disability status, sexual orientation, and gender identity affect virtually every aspect of life for emerging adults (Leiner et al., 2018) including educational/ employment opportunities, income, health care access, and overall well-being. Unfortunately, young adults are particularly vulnerable to discrimination, in that they have fewer coping skills relative to their elder cohorts. Because emerging adulthood is such a critical period of development, the impact of racism and discrimination can have lifelong consequences. Young adults who frequently experience discrimination are at risk for both mental and physical health issues. Racism has been shown to increase stress levels, which can lead to a weakened immune system and elevated blood pressure. A relationship has been shown between discrimination and both substance misuse and unhealthy eating; sleep may also be affected. Depression, anxiety, and other forms of emotional distress in emerging adults are also associated with racism and discrimination (Lewsley & Slater, 2020).

Legal Issues and Deepening Political Divisions

In the politically divisive climate in which we currently live, legal threats to individual freedoms are cause for concern for both parents and their adult children. The decision of the U.S. Supreme Court to overturn a woman's right to abortion has and will likely continue in the future to contribute to feelings of anxiety and uncertainty among emerging adults. Young adults, especially those with financial constraints and limited mobility, are particularly at risk for disruption in career and educational goals as well as financial instability in the face of an unintended pregnancy. Today's parents feel worried and anxious for their children with respect to their physical and emotional health and safety as a result of this uncertainty (Clay, 2024). The Supreme Court's decision regarding abortion may be just the beginning of a broader change in civil rights given our current political landscape. Other vulnerable areas identified by legal experts include same-sex marriage, the separation of church and state, and the repeal of affirmative action at universities. Changes in any of these areas could further limit the rights of all citizens, including emerging adults and their parents and subsequently increase anxiety.

In addition, legal threats to the LGBTQ community are of great concern. LGBTQ young adults have been victimized by the recent efforts of some political factions to either restrict existing educational policies and legal protections for LGBTQ children and adults and/or enact other discriminatory legislation against them (e.g., bans against LGBT-related books, transgender access to public bathrooms that corresponds to gender identity, and exemptions of LGBT antidiscrimination laws based on religious beliefs). Such political efforts have led to fear and confusion for both young adults and their parents (Abreu, Sostre, Gonzalez, Lockett, & Matsuno, 2022; Abreu, Sostre, Gonzalez, Lockett, Matsuno, & Mosley, 2022). And controversy surrounding the needs of gender nonconforming youth has contributed to even more anxiety for parents and for emerging adults themselves.

Changes in Substance Use Behaviors

Young adults typically experiment with substances while they explore their identities. Emerging adults may resort to a variety of substances, some legal and some not, in an effort both to fit in with peers and to self-medicate anxiety and stress. This, coupled with recent cultural and legislative changes, has, for example, resulted in a substantial increase in nicotine vaping and marijuana use. The recreational use of cannabis is now legal in 21 states, and its medical use is legalized in 38 states and the District of Columbia. The ease of accessibility, the evolution of alternate inhalational methods (e.g., processed cannabis vaping liquids and oils composed of chemical agents such as flavoring substances), and targeted marketing campaigns have contributed to a rise in popularity of these substances among young adults. The use of both cannabis and nicotine has progressively increased in young adults (National Institute on Drug Abuse, 2018, 2020, 2022). Prolonged use of these substances can contribute to medical problems including bronchitis symptoms; e-cigarette and vaping–associated lung injury, also known as the EVALI syndrome; cavities; seizures; heart disease; and cancer. Cannabis misuse can also impact areas of the brain integral to its development and to neurological functioning (e.g., memory, attention) in adolescents and young adults whose brains have not completely matured.

The use of prescription opioids (e.g., oxycodone, codeine, hydromorphone, morphine) among adolescents and young adults has skyrocketed into an epidemic in recent years. Many begin their use with a prescription for pain, perhaps due to a sports injury or having wisdom teeth pulled, and some will continue on using to medicate anxiety or other forms of distress. For some young adults, this pattern can eventually lead to illicit opioid use (Guarino et al., 2018; McCabe et al., 2021). The entrance of fentanyl and other potent synthetic drugs is very scary. These dangerous drugs sometimes masquerade as colorful candies and are readily available on the internet. Even one-time use of these drugs can lead to death.

Social Media

Although social media has its positive aspects (e.g., it offers a forum for maintaining contact with friends and family), it is also believed to have a negative impact on the mental health of today's teens and young adults (Ilakkuvan et al., 2019). Social media leads young people to compare themselves with idealized images of their peers. They can keep track of their friends, know where they are, and who is interacting with whom. They also know when they are being left out (Perrine, 2022). Many adolescents and young adults use social media to connect and to address isolation and loneliness, but unfortunately the result is often anxiety and depression.

Another negative use of social media is cyberbullying, defined as the intentional use of smart phones, computers, and other electronic devices to inflict harm on others. Cyberbullying, unlike the more traditional bullying, is difficult to escape because cyberbullies can maintain an online presence 24/7. Additionally, the negative and hurtful posts aimed at the target go viral and are likely to remain both permanent and public. Probably the most troubling aspect of cyberbullying is the capacity to be anonymous, which makes it challenging to detect the source.

COVID-19

The COVID pandemic brought challenges to all of us. Although health professionals have suggested that some young adults were less prone to experience COVID-19 infections than others, infection rates alone fail to account for the psychological impact of COVID-19 on emerging adults (Keeter, 2021). Their already-uncertain future became even more precarious; autonomy and self-directedness were reduced. Emerging adulthood, a phase of life typically bursting with choices and options, became a time full of constraints. Many young adults also lost their jobs, exacerbating their economic insecurity.

Many colleges and universities temporarily closed, while others transitioned to virtual-only courses in an effort to stop or slow the spread of COVID-19. This sudden move to online learning platforms had a profound impact on emerging adults by limiting their opportunities for stimulation and social interaction. Social distancing was required; this, combined with online learning, contributed to isolation and boredom, which led to the heightened use of social media.

In addition to emerging adults becoming reliant on social media to cope with the many unwelcome changes brought on by COVID-19, many also began to use and misuse substances. Patterns of and motives for substance use among young adults during the COVID-19 pandemic appeared to shift as young adults drank alcohol more frequently, but consumed less alcohol per occasion, and their use was motivated by a desire to cope with distress rather than for social enhancement and conformity (Graupensperger et al., 2021).

Other fallout from the COVID-19 pandemic includes widespread racial prejudice, discrimination, and hate crimes against people of Asian descent (e.g., Croucher et al., 2020; Hahm et al., 2021). This anti-Asian sentiment is particularly visible on social media and has resulted in many Asians fearing for their lives. This has led to increased alcohol consumption among young adults of Asian descent as a coping strategy (Keum & Choi, 2022). In addition, what started as a public health crisis evolved into a highly polarizing and politicized issue that further divided people and created mistrust of the medical profession.

Loneliness

We would be remiss if we did not address the pervasive feelings of loneliness and isolation that were, and to some degree remain, a part of the emerging adult experience at present. The COVID-19 pandemic certainly contributed to these feelings, forcing young adults into isolation for health and safety reasons. Although social media helped to fill the gap in social connectedness for many young adults, for others it magnified feelings of loneliness and social inadequacy. There is growing acknowledgment, as evidenced by the Office of the Surgeon General (2023) report, that loneliness is an epidemic, especially among young adults. The physical and mental health consequences of social isolation (e.g., sleep problems, inflammation and immune changes, depression, anxiety, addiction, suicidality, and self-harm) are deeply worrisome.

PSYCHOLOGICAL DISTRESS IN YOUNG ADULTS: ANOTHER PANDEMIC?

Perhaps the stones in the road we've just discussed contribute to the mental health crisis raging in the lives of young people today. Many children, adolescents, and young adults are struggling with depression, self-injury, suicide attempts, and completed suicides

(Abramson, 2022). Well-publicized proclamations and funding initiatives (e.g., increase in mental health providers in schools, implementing 24/7 crisis hotline, expanding access to out-of-school programs) have been offered to address these concerns, especially in the pre-K–12 environment (U.S. Department of Education, 2022).

As a parent you may have had access to various services for children and adolescents. However, when your child turns 18, the situation changes drastically. Because it is easier to study college students, most of the research focuses on this population. Two key studies report compelling results. For example, one survey of 350,000 students at more than 350 campuses (Lipson et al., 2022) found that the mental health of college students across the United States has been on a steady decline from 2013 to 2021, with an overall 135% increase in depression symptoms and a 110% rise in anxiety symptoms during that period. In another national survey, almost three quarters of students reported moderate or severe psychological distress (American College Health Association, 2022). At the same time, it is important to note that more than half of emerging adults who may be experiencing anxiety and depression are not enrolled in postsecondary education (Hanson, 2022). Regardless of their pathway after high school, the severity of symptoms for anxiety and depression in this age group increased steadily over the past decade and hit a new high during the COVID outbreak (Kujawa et al., 2020).

This mental health pandemic among young adults began on a collision course with what is commonly regarded as a broken mental health care system. Mental health care in America continues to be stymied by multiple challenges, including chronic underfunding, widespread provider shortages, insufficient hospital or residential beds, too few options for intermediate care, and a lack of integrated services including affordable housing specifically for persons with mental health disorders. News headlines document serious injury and death of young persons with mental illness at the hands of untrained police officers. In many cases, disastrous consequences occur when first responders, such as police officers, are called to the scene without the necessary training to manage mental health crises appropriately. Left without adequate support and services, the depressed, anxious, and otherwise distressed adolescent is poorly equipped to handle the challenges of becoming an emerging adult.

The Health Insurance Portability and Accountability Act (HIPAA) was created with the purpose of protecting patients' medical information from being shared without their knowledge or permission. This means that all young adults, beginning at age 18, are able to make their own health care decisions including medical procedures, medications, and other treatments. You, as a parent, are no longer in the driver's seat regarding medical and mental health care decisions for your young adult, nor are you able to access your adult child's medical information without their written consent. Your adult child's medical records are private, even if your child is still under your health insurance. We discuss the implications of HIPAA for you and your adult child in more detail in Chapter 6.

ARE PARENTS OF TODAY'S EMERGING ADULTS OVERSTRESSED?

The chaotic and unpredictable nature of life in the United States has contributed to significant stress for parents. Such parental stress leads to anxiety, which often manifests in the tendency to "overparent"— that is, hovering over their young adult and trying to ensure their well-being. Overprotection is a natural response when parents feel uncertain and fearful. The term *helicopter parenting* was first introduced in the early 1990s and has gained tremendous traction over time; it is characterized by overinvolvement, overprotection, and even overcontrol. Although this label can apply to parents of children of any age, it has been widely applied to parents of young adults (e.g., parents accompany adult children to university interviews, attend discussions with tutors about grades or progress, or insert themselves into their young adult's job application process and workplace relations).

Although the constant hovering may heighten parents' sense of security regarding their young adult's safety and "good" choices, it also serves to shield the young adult from failure experiences and any associated negative emotions. On the surface, this may seem like a win–win, but let's look a bit closer at this situation. When an adult child has not had the prior experience of "failure," how do they learn to deal with the bumps in the road? If they have never been allowed to fall down, skin their knees, and get back up, how do they learn to be resilient—or, for that matter, learn that they are capable of getting back up again?

For some parents, hovering behaviors with their adult child may indicate a concern for how the young adult's actions reflect on the parents. It can further serve to protect the parent's "reputation" by ensuring the "right" choices and the "right behaviors" from their young adult. Regardless of the type of concern behind the hovering behavior, the likely outcome of helicopter parenting is a cohort of young adults lacking in self-efficacy as well as the ability to function independently. Inadequate coping skills and vulnerability to depression and anxiety are also challenges for this population (Bradley-Geist & Olson-Buchanan, 2014; Rettner, 2010).

Clearly our world has become much more complex, and the stakes of "letting go" of your young adult appear to be higher. Although parents are constantly being encouraged to take the bubble wrap off their children and let them learn from their mistakes and disappointments, it can be frightening and quite difficult to do so. But while letting go of helicopter parenting is stressful, so is continuing to practice it. Helicopter parenting requires constant vigilance, which is emotionally and physically exhausting and puts you in a state of chronic stress.

In addition to persistent worry about their young adults, today's parents must also contend with financial concerns about rising food prices, higher housing costs, and increased barriers to health care. It is not surprising, given these stressors, that many parents report their own symptoms of anxiety and depression as well as a sense of apathy, lethargy, and fatigue. Therefore, learning strategies to manage chronic levels of stress is imperative at this point in your journey.

YOUR FIRST AND MOST IMPORTANT TOOL: BREATHING TO CALM DOWN

Given all the stressors that today's emerging adults face, it's no wonder that many parents today experience worry and concern about their young adults. It is essential for parents to appreciate the degree to which this chronic stress can have a negative impact on their adult children on a physiological and emotional level. It is also important for you, the reader, to understand the impact of stress on your physical and mental well-being. Throughout this book, we'll be reminding you to breathe.

Imagine the following scenario: You are taking a walk on a cool autumn day down the sunny path in the woods near your home. As you round the bend in the path, you suddenly come face to face with a 500-pound black bear! Immediately your breathing is shallow and rapid, your heart races, your blood pressure skyrockets, your pupils dilate, and your muscles tense. These changes in your body's functioning are what is known as the stress response, also known as fight–flight–freeze. Although these bodily changes may be frightening to experience, they are the body's way of protecting itself and they have allowed humans to survive for centuries. Unfortunately, the body is unable to distinguish between a life-threatening stressor and a minor day-to-day stressor, such as failure to pay a bill, and this often allows us to become victims of false alarms.

Let's take a quick look at what happens in your brain and ultimately your body when you are under stress and/or highly anxious.

This statement may prompt you to wonder how having such an understanding could be of benefit to you. The short answer is easy: Knowledge is power! Once you understand that your brain is doing what it is supposed to do to keep you safe, your fear will begin to ease, and you'll feel empowered to practice the calming exercises you will learn in this book. Here we offer a brief discussion about the four parts of the brain involved in the stress response: the amygdala, hypothalamus, hippocampus, and the cerebral cortex. Figure 1.1 depicts these parts of the brain.

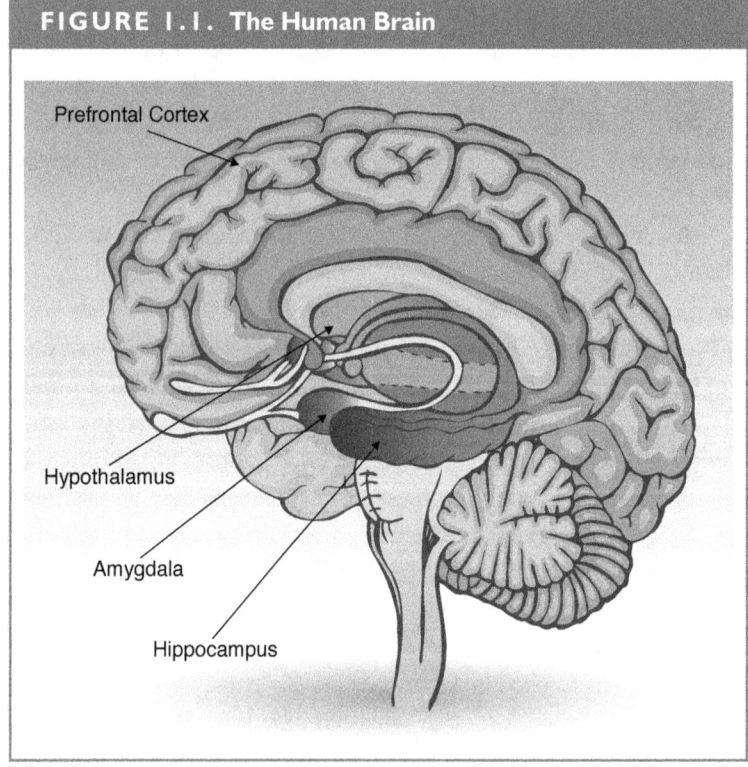

FIGURE 1.1. The Human Brain

We will begin with the amygdala, or the alarm center. When a threat is perceived, the amygdala immediately sends a distress signal to the hypothalamus, or the command center, telling it to alert the rest of the body that danger is present! The hypothalamus directs the sympathetic nervous system, or the body's accelerator, to pump hormones into the bloodstream. These hormones work together to deliver stored sugar and fat into your bloodstream giving your body a burst of energy—that is, all the scary symptoms—to do what is necessary to fight or flee from the threat.

The hippocampus, or the recorder, is busy keeping a log of information about the current threat as well as highly charged emotional life experiences from the past. Additionally, the hippocampus records our successful and unsuccessful attempts to cope with these scary experiences from the past so that we learn from them. The cerebral cortex, or the CEO of the brain, is responsible for executive functioning—for example, planning, organizing, and problem-solving. The cerebral cortex reviews the current threat as well as past memories and then determines a path forward. In so doing, it works with the parasympathetic nervous system, or the brakes, to slow our bodies down.

Chronic stress can keep the amygdala activated and our bodies on high alert. It's like a siren that never shuts off, and the result is an overload of stress hormones that keep your body pumped up and struggling to return to a relaxed state. Whether you are experiencing a life-altering event, a high level of chronic stress, or a daily annoyance, your goal is to learn how to communicate with the cerebral cortex and the brakes of the nervous system. The most efficient way to do this is to focus on your breath.

Deep breathing, also known as diaphragmatic or belly breathing, is the best and most efficient way to slow the body down. Belly breathing involves taking a deep breath through your nose and slowly releasing it through your mouth. As you breathe in, put your hand on your belly and imagine it blowing up like a balloon; as you exhale, slowly let the balloon deflate. Breathing deeply increases the supply of oxygen to your brain which in turn activates the body's brakes, or the parasympathetic nervous system. Once the brakes are activated, your heart rate slows, your muscles relax, and your blood pressure decreases allowing your body to reach a state of calmness. Deep breathing is one of the most effective strategies for managing stress and anxiety.

Belly breathing and cyclic sighing, described subsequently, seem to be very simple behaviors, yet they carry a powerful punch against runaway stress. When we are in the whirlpool of stress, it's all but impossible to engage in anything but survival mode tactics. We don't think straight, and our ability to have meaningful discussions with our young adults, and anyone else for that matter, is severely impaired. Learning to slow down this runaway stress train by using breathing behaviors allows us to get ready to listen to our young adults at a deeper, more effective level. We have included a breathing exercise here for you to try. See Exhibit 1.1.

We also recommend a technique called cyclic sighing (see Exhibit 1.2). Evidence suggests that cyclic sighing is even more beneficial than mindfulness meditation in decreasing anxiety and improving mood (Balban et al., 2023). Because this is also especially difficult to do in the heat of the moment, we recommend regular practice of this during periods of relative calm.

EXHIBIT 1.1. Calming Exercise: 4-7-8 Breathing

- Completely exhale through your mouth.
- Close your mouth and inhale through your nose to the count of four.
- Hold your breath to the count of seven.
- Exhale to the count of eight.
- Repeat three times.

EXHIBIT 1.2. Calming Exercise: Cyclic Sighing

- Breathe in through your nose until your lungs are comfortably full.
- Take another, but deeper sip of air, to expand your lungs even more.
- Slowly exhale through your mouth.
- For full benefit, repeat these steps for about 5 minutes.

SUMMARY

Whew! No wonder you are feeling unsettled, confused, and perhaps a bit anxious! All the volatility and uncertainty swirling around in our environment today has us struggling to find solid ground and choose a path forward with our parenting responsibilities. The many factors that influence our children on their journey to adulthood can overwhelm our sense of stability and complicate our role as parents. In this chapter, we provided a picture of the normative process of emerging adulthood as a time of instability, exploration, and self-focus. We described the current chaotic environment in which we live as well as the "stones" that make emerging adulthood even more daunting. It is important for you as a parent to keep in mind that your adult child's journey can be rocky in the best of circumstances. The uncertainty of our world, greater social isolation, increased violence, natural and human-made disasters, among other realities, all highlight the significant vulnerabilities for emerging adults in terms of developing symptoms of anxiety, depression, and other emotional distress. Not surprisingly, emerging adults reported increases in symptoms of anxiety and depression as well as fear and stress during COVID-19.

In Chapter 2, we consider the effects of all the chaos in the world on you as a parent and explore the normative challenges of parenting young adults in such a context. We encourage you to gain a new perspective on your role as a parent by suggesting relevant parenting information together with useful strategies to pivot from primary caretaker to "coach." Our intent is to support you in making this necessary shift.

POINTS TO POCKET

- Times are truly volatile, uncertain, and chaotic. We need new tools for this journey. Read on.
- Adulting is a complex and extended process today. Some young adults may take additional time before making decisions regarding marriage and childbearing, and ultimately experience greater happiness and satisfaction with their choices.
- Breathing is the most essential tool for managing your own anxiety as you manage the stress associated with your adult child's passage through emerging adulthood.
- Many young adults are stuck and overwhelmed. This is quite common and doesn't necessarily mean that your young adult is stuck in your house forever!
- Don't blow a fuse! Many emerging adults experience deficits in administrative skills. However, your young adult can still move successfully through emerging adulthood.
- Einstein said the definition of insanity is doing the same thing over and over and expecting different results. To survive as a parent today you need new skills and a new perspective. Same old, same old will not cut it!

CHAPTER 2

THE PIVOTS BEGIN

Parents can only give good advice or put them on the right path but the final forming of a person's character lies in their own hands.

—Anne Frank, *The Diary of a Young Girl*

In Chapter 1, you learned about the process of emerging adulthood as well as its many challenges and stumbling blocks, all of which can feel overwhelming. We further conveyed the complexity of the process as we examined the tasks of emerging adulthood in the context of our current VUCA (volatile, uncertain, complex, and ambiguous) world.

Before we pivot toward the coach role, let's consider what an effective caretaker does. In that role, you have communicated effectively with your child, which also involves helping them to understand and name their feelings. You have set boundaries, provided direction and consistency, and fostered autonomy; you were flexible and responsive to their needs; and kept them safe. In addition, your own self-care required your attention. That's quite a hefty load to carry. These are the foundational skills you will build on with each of the next three pivots. For example, setting boundaries with your toddler perhaps involved childproofing your home environment and not giving in to tantrums; boundaries with adolescents and young adults are no less important. We explore boundaries with young adults in more detail as we pivot toward the role of coach. Although it was and continues to be important to recognize your own needs in the process, it's no wonder that your self-care may have been short-changed or neglected.

In this chapter, we focus on you as you pivot from caretaker to coach in our current world of chaos and unpredictability. We discuss how the new role of coach might look for you. This pivot likely poses one of the biggest challenges for parents of emerging adults; it may feel considerably different from your other pivots and, in reality, it is. There is more of a letting go in this pivot, as well as a redefinition of your role. This may sound simple; it is not. The tools offered in this chapter will not only build confidence in your role as coach, they will also put you on much firmer ground in relating to and helping your young adult through the rough waters they encounter.

THE PIVOT FROM CARETAKER TO COACH

When you hear the word *coach*, what comes to mind? What constitutes coaching behavior, and how is it different from being a caretaker? In many ways, the role of a coach involves a step back from "doing for" your adult child. You are still very much present but sitting in the passenger's seat rather than behind the wheel. A coach is empathic and a good listener; they model desired behavior and respond to questions. They also teach and give feedback to their young adult. Like any good coach, the parent in "coach mode" makes recommendations to their young adult, but it is up to that young adult to carry out the actions on their own, regardless of your apprehension. The job of coach is actually more complex than that of caretaker because you are constantly walking a very fine line. You need to anticipate when to back off and distance yourself, and that is not always obvious.

During the pivot to coach, you officially hand the keys to your young adult, climb out of the driver's seat of their lives, and move into copilot mode. From this vantage point, you teach, or model, skills and offer encouragement; you don't do for them anymore, but you will show them how to do for themselves.

Let's consider this example to illustrate how the role of coach differs from that of caretaker. Your young adult calls to say they just finished final exams and wants to spend the next week and a half relaxing with their friends who have rented a house at the beach. As you talk with them, it becomes clear that they don't have the $500 to pay for their share of the trip or any money for food. It is also clear from recent conversations with them that they have made some unwise decisions regarding their monthly expenses (e.g., Uber Eats 5 nights a week, computer games and other luxuries they absolutely "needed"). They really want to go to the beach and come to you begging for financial help. As a caretaker, you can easily be pulled into their excitement and agree to pay all or most of their expenses. Afterall, they just finished a rough semester. Although this takes care of the immediate situation, it also hinders your young adult's ability to learn how to take care of their money issues in the long run.

As you pivot toward coach, you see the opportunity for a teachable moment. First you consider your child's psychological distress and their level of functioning in this situation (refer to Figures 2 and 3 in this book's Introduction). As a coach, you understand that while your young adult is upset and perhaps even angry at the situation, they are also functioning well enough to be able to take in what you have to show them. You empathize with their wanting to go to the beach and at the same time let them experience the consequences of their spending habits and the resulting disappointment at losing out on the trip this time around. You must be strategic in how you approach them, and you are looking for cues that your young adult can listen to what you have to say and take some direction. When the time is right, you and your young adult will sit down together with paper and pencil, and you will teach them how to set up a budget so they can plan for the recurring expenses every month. Periodically you will check in to see how things are going with their budget.

When is the right time to pivot from caretaker to coach? Generally speaking, once your child reaches age 18, it is best to shift away from the caretaker role when possible, although you may need to pivot back to that role if your young adult is in severe distress and functioning at a minimal level. The coach role is appropriate when your young adult is moderately distressed and somewhat low functioning.

Let's consider another example of the pivot from caretaker to coach by returning to Claire's story about her daughter, Anne. As you read, take time to reflect on the emotional struggles often characteristic of the pivot from caretaker to coach:

> When Anne told me she wanted to switch her major from history to biology because she was bored, my first reaction was, "Oh no! Here we go again!" She had a habit of quitting activities or other commitments, like trumpet lessons, as soon as she lost interest. And she lost interest for a variety of reasons— the lessons demanded too much, the practices were too long, she didn't have any friends there, and so on. While I wanted Anne to enjoy whatever she chose to do, I also felt she needed to follow through with her commitments, since quitting isn't always an option in the game of life. I knew a biology major would be more difficult for Anne given her learning disability; I was worried she was setting herself up either to lose interest or, even worse, to feel overwhelmed and inadequate. Anne was very bright, but her learning disability often led her to doubt her academic ability. It was troubling to see Anne's self-confidence ebb away during her later teenage and young adult years. I was also annoyed and frustrated when she refused to request academic accommodations that would have put her on equal footing with her peers. As much as she wanted to succeed, it seemed she wanted to fit in more; that meant no accommodations. I tried repeatedly to talk with Anne about how the accommodations could help her succeed, but I might as well have been talking to the wall.

What is your reaction to Claire's story? Does it sound familiar to you? Claire is clearly worried about her daughter and confused about how best to respond. It is easy to understand how many parents, in Claire's position, might overact. However, overfunctioning or helicoptering as a parent of a young adult is ill advised. Claire's task here is to determine how to relate to Anne without further eroding her self-confidence and fostering her dependence on her and Stan. Remember, effective parenting at any age requires engaging in behaviors that foster your child's autonomy. This is a great example of how difficult it is to make a decision regarding which role is most appropriate at this point in time. Anne appears to be at a low or moderate level of distress, and she seems to be functioning fairly well. Claire, however, is concerned that her daughter doesn't really understand the possible ramifications of her decision. Instead, she is following her pattern of impulsively jumping into something new because she's bored.

For so many parents like Claire, sitting back and watching their young adults make questionable decisions and derail their plans is very difficult. And yet, when your young adult turns 18, that magical number, they are considered legal adults, and you are no longer the one making the decisions. This is a hard place for many of us as parents to be. We know from our own personal and professional experiences how to navigate difficult circumstances, and yet our young adults cannot or will not listen to us. We struggle as parents with letting them make their own mistakes and worry that some of those mistakes could deter both their immediate and long-term plans. We have to shift our thinking from being a caretaker (stepping in and doing things for our young adult) to being a coach (instructing them how to do things for themselves), and that is a difficult process for many of us. Let's take a look at the pivot you are heading into as you move toward the role of coach.

Returning to our example, Claire is feeling more and more frustrated with Anne's tentativeness about getting accommodations.

How might Claire approach Anne in a coaching mode? As a coach, Claire might validate and empathize with the challenge of asking for help. She might need to point out that Anne's learning disability does not define who she is; the learning disability is only one aspect of her. She might also note that getting extra time on tests does not constitute a special advantage but merely puts her on equal footing with her peers. To be an effective coach, Claire first needs to understand the university's requirements and procedures for requesting learning accommodations. Because she has been through the testing and accommodation procedures when Anne was younger, she has some familiarity with the process. Claire searches on the university's website under the umbrella of student services. As she reviews the requirements that are necessary to request accommodations, she develops a tentative action plan to help her daughter understand and navigate the university's process. She will need to engage Anne in a calm, nonthreatening manner and share what she has learned. Together, they can create a step-by-step plan that Anne can follow— for example, scheduling an appointment, gathering necessary paperwork such as documentation of the learning disability, and making a list of questions to ask at the meeting. Although Claire is instrumental in helping Anne figure out what to do, it is up to Anne to put the plan in motion.

 ## THE COACH SKILL SET

Let's consider the unique skills of a coach which allow Claire to be more effective with Anne. See Exhibit 2.1.

Listen Intently

The heart and soul of all effective communication is listening. In her book *The Zen of Listening*, Shafir (2003) maintained that people

---

> **EXHIBIT 2.1.   How to Be an Effective Coach for Your Young Adult**
>
> - Listen intently.
> - Validate emotions.
> - Employ empathy.
> - Use clear, deliberate communication.
> - Use open-ended questions and statements.
> - Use emotion regulation.
> - Set and maintain your own personal boundaries.
> - Support autonomy.
> - Do self-care.

spend 40% of waking hours in a day listening and that most retain only 25% of what is said within minutes of listening. How can this be? One reason is the internal chatter in our heads, such as self-critical thoughts or even running down our to-do list while trying to listen to the speaker. Another reason is the many external distractions including cell phones, radio, and television, among others. To tune out internal and external noise, Shafir suggested putting ourselves in the other person's "movie." Think about sitting in a theater and becoming absorbed in the story on the screen. Your mouth is shut, and your ears are open, and your attention is fully given over to what you are hearing and seeing. Another way to understand this is to think about a time recently when you were talking and the other person wasn't listening. How did you know they weren't listening? What did that feel like? Now think of a time when you were listened to. How did you know you were heard and what did that feel like? Being fully present in this way is one of the greatest gifts one person can give to another. Listening is a skill that can be learned and strengthened over time.

Listening intently is a whole-body experience involving the ears, eyes, mind, and heart. Thus, when we listen to our young adult in the role of coach, we are better able to connect with the person we're listening to on an emotional level, not just the rational or logical level. Shafir (2003) approaches listening as a mindset that entails attending to the present moment; quieting your own mind; observing a person's words, tone of voice, facial expression, and body language; and tuning in to your mind as well. In essence, Shafir emphasized the importance of paying attention to nonverbal as well as verbal communication. Facial expression, body language, and tone of voice are all forms of nonverbal communication. It might be surprising to learn that as much as 80% to 90% of meaning comes from nonverbal rather than verbal communication. This highlights the importance of attending to all aspects of communication, not just what is said.

Listening intently allows Claire as coach to connect with Anne in a way that makes ongoing communication possible as well as being able to teach Anne how to prepare herself to ask for help. Claire listened intently as Anne told her about how anxious she felt at the prospect of going to the student services office for help. She could see an opening to show her daughter how she might approach the visit. They both sat down, took some deep breaths, and started to establish a plan for how Anne would move forward.

Validate Emotions

So what do we mean by validate? At a very basic level, we are saying that you acknowledge the feeling, help your young adult label it, and then use the experience of that emotion to teach them how to cope with their feelings and to problem solve. In our experience, we have found many parents have difficulties dealing with their children's emotions, and this intensifies as their children become young adults. For many of us, this was not the norm when we were growing up. If you didn't experience emotion-focused parenting yourself, you may find this quite challenging. Beginning in the late 1990s, psychologists and child development experts stressed the need for parents to attend fully to and validate their child's feelings. This is now considered a fundamental skill for effective caretaking (Eisenberg et al., 1998; Gottman, 1998; Gottman et al., 1996; Havighurst et al., 2020). When we validate our child's or young adult's emotions, we are adopting Daniel Goleman's (2005) concept of *emotional intelligence*, or EQ. Simply stated, emotional intelligence is the ability to be aware of and manage your own feelings, and the ability to understand how another person might feel (also known as empathy). Goleman emphasized the importance of parents facilitating emotional intelligence in their children because children with a high EQ tend to perform well in school, have better mental health, and grow to be successful adults. Ideally, parents begin fostering EQ in their children from an early age.

In his book, *Raising an Emotionally Intelligent Child: The Heart of Parenting*, Dr. John Gottman (1998) also emphasized the critical role the child's emotions can play when one is learning to parent effectively. He observed that some parents respond to their young children by dismissing, ignoring, and/or minimizing their child's feelings. Other parents may disapprove, judge, or criticize the child's feelings. Regardless, these parents believe the expression of emotions is a sign of weakness or at least being unproductive. Gottman stressed the importance of validating their feelings and teaching them to label their emotions. Parents can use their child's expression of negative emotion (anger, sadness, grief, jealousy, etc.) as a teaching moment. They listen to and empathize with their child; they do not minimize the feeling or degrade their child for experiencing any emotion. Once the parent validates their child's negative feelings, they encourage the child to think about what such emotions may be telling them.

Although Goleman and Gottman wrote primarily about emotional intelligence/emotion focused parenting with children, we include it here because it is an important skill for parents of young adults in psychological distress. Their recommendations encourage parents to begin conversations with their distressed young adults by focusing on their emotions. Remember, if you were not raised to understand and constructively manage your emotions, this can be especially challenging. If this is the case, you and your young adult may be trying to learn the same set of skills. It is important for you as a parent to be comfortable with your own emotions to be able to handle the emotional ups and downs of your young adult. It is also essential to remember that this is a learning process that gradually takes shape as you pivot from caretaker to coach.

Employ Empathy

Closely aligned with validation of your young adult's emotions is the skill of empathy. Simply put, empathy is the ability to put yourself in another person's shoes, to understand what they are experiencing from their perspective, even if you've never had the experience yourself. There is a difference between empathy and sympathy. When you empathize with someone, you put yourself in their shoes and understand as much as you can what they are experiencing while maintaining a clear sense of being separate from them. You also leave intact their sense of agency—their ability to act for themselves. When you sympathize, you not only put yourself in their shoes, but you walk around in them, and the distinction between the two of you becomes less clear. Sympathy also involves the implicit notion that they can't take care of themselves, so someone else must do it for them. Such a message serves to reduce their sense of agency. Empathy is closely aligned with effective listening because both require being fully present with the other person. Both empathy and listening are critical skills for parents to use to communicate with their children at any age—and most particularly, their young adults.

Empathy is not an easy thing to embody, especially when you are under stress. In fact, it might be the last thing on your mind as you interact with your young adult. To empathize, you need to engage both your heart and your mind, not an easy thing to do when you feel distressed. And yet, it is doable. Take a step back, listen to your young adult, and focus on the situation from their point of view. What are they trying to tell you? If you can check your own feelings and immediate urge to respond from your own perspective, you will more fully understand what they need you to hear.

As Claire listened to Anne describe her feelings and rationale for not seeking help for her learning disability, she realized that she and Anne viewed Anne's learning disability very differently. Claire was able to put aside her own perception and respond to her daughter with empathy.

> What I hear you saying, Anne, is that you don't want to be different from anyone else in the class. You feel embarrassed that you have to ask for help. Does that make sense to you?

By asking Anne if she heard her accurately, Claire is likely gaining further clarity and demonstrating her respect for Anne's autonomy. Like Claire, you can use the tools of listening intently and empathizing to lower the temperature in the room and open the door to effective communication even with the more difficult dialogues.

Use Clear, Deliberate Communication

As a coach for your young adult, you may need to alter the way you communicate with them. The way you communicated as a caretaker is not the most effective way to communicate as a coach. Integral to effective communication are reasonable expectations for where your adult child is on their developmental journey. It's easy to want to compare where they are in the process with your own transition to adulthood. Don't do this. Today's young adults are living in a society considerably different from the one in which you grew up.

A close relationship with your emerging adult is possible only when communication is healthy and mutually respectful. As a coach, you want to demonstrate respect by inviting discussion; talking, not lecturing; asking open-ended questions; attending to tone of voice and body language; and believing your young adult is capable of moving forward in their life development (McNulty, 2021).

Exhibit 2.2 contains a list of rules to help you communicate effectively with your young adult in your role as coach. Many of

---

EXHIBIT 2.2. Rules for Clear, Deliberate Communication

- Monitor your own air time. As a coach, talk less and listen more.
- Seek first to understand. Attend to and understand your young adult before adding your perspective.
- Speak from your own experience (e.g., "I feel" vs. "You make me feel").
- Follow the "XYZ" formula: "I feel X, when you do Y, in situation Z" (e.g., "I felt frustrated when you didn't mail that letter yesterday after you agreed to do so").
- Avoid absolutes. The words "always" and "never" are not accurate and invite an argument.
- Stay in your own lane. Remember that you can only change your own actions and perspectives; you can't control your young adult.
- Do not collect stamps. Keeping score of past hurts in your relationship with your young adult and/or holding grudges helps no one.
- Focus on solving the problem, not who is at fault.
- When things heat up, take a time-out. Then come back together when you have both cooled off.
- When others make requests of you, allow yourself to think it over. Give yourself permission not to answer immediately.

---

these are intuitive and may fit comfortably with what you already do. These rules are also helpful with other family members. Please note that in times of stress it is easy to forget them.

Use Open-Ended Questions and Statements

Part of being able to communicate clearly is knowing how to make strategic use of questions. Most of us use questions too frequently in communicating with others, especially when we are stressed out or don't know what to say. So often when we find ourselves in emotionally charged situations, we tend to fire off what are known as closed questions, those questions that require a one-word response ("yes" or "no") and effectively shut down communication. For example, your daughter comes by after work and tells you she's applied for a third job to speed up the process of getting a car. She is already working 50 hours a week and has almost no time for herself. You know how stress affects her, and you kind of lose it. "Are you crazy?! Where did you get this idea? Do you really think you can fit another job into your schedule?" A reaction like this will only push your daughter away and cut off the conversation.

Open-ended questions, by contrast, invite the young adult to share more of what they are thinking and feeling. A coach would likely ask an open-ended question such as, "What do you find appealing about this choice?" or, alternatively, make a statement like "Help me understand what you find appealing about this choice," or "Tell me more about what you are thinking," giving the young adult plenty of room to respond in their own way. You get more information, and they feel heard. Let's return to the previous example. This time, you take a breath and then respond as a coach: "Wow, that's going to leave you with even less free time. Help me understand where you're going to find the time for the new job."

As you are practicing clear and deliberate communication, remember to monitor your own emotions and manage them productively. In using these new skills, you will undoubtedly make mistakes. And when you do, take the time to apologize. An apology can go a long way toward establishing a close connection with your emerging adult.

Use Emotion Regulation

Emotion regulation is another skill integral to a successful pivot to the role of coach. The term refers to the ability to control your emotion so you can express that emotion constructively, honestly, and in a way that is in line with your goals and values. Communication of emotion in healthy ways can lead to higher quality social relationships as well as improved overall functioning. Perhaps you feel confident in your ability to manage your emotions; if so, regard this as a review or reminder. On the other hand, if you have experienced situations in which controlling your emotions was difficult or challenging, consider employing the following skills to assist you in more effectively managing or controlling your emotions. In the example with Claire, she demonstrated emotion regulation when she practiced deep breathing.

You may want to take a moment to "ground" yourself when you become aware of intense or overwhelming emotion. Grounding helps keep you in the present moment. It is an essential skill for you to use on bad days, during frustrating moments, and, most of all, when you find yourself experiencing high levels of stress and anxiety. One of the most effective grounding exercises makes use of your five senses (see Exhibit 2.3).

Once you are grounded, the next step is to recognize and name the emotion(s) you are experiencing. Remember that your feelings don't define you. They do, however, provide you with important

EXHIBIT 2.3. Calming Exercise: Grounding Using Your Senses

- Take a deep breath.
- Look around and name five things you can see.
- Look around and name four things you can hear.
- Name three things you can touch.
- Name two things you can smell.
- Name one thing you can taste.

information about yourself. When you experience difficulty clarifying your feelings, sensations in your body may be helpful. The crucial thing is to be as open, curious, and nonjudgmental toward your own emotions as you are about your emerging adult's feelings. In Claire's case, she feels increasingly frustrated when Anne refuses to ask for accommodations for her learning disability. Her heart rate increases and her breathing gets shallow as she starts imagining her daughter never getting her act together. She needs to take another couple of deep breaths and consider what's going on. She realizes that this may be the first time she "can't fix Anne," and if she's not careful, she could conclude that she has failed as a mother. See Exhibit 2.4 for a list of skills to assist you in regulating your emotions.

Claire is beginning to realize that there is a connection among her physical sensations, thoughts, and feelings. Claire's ability to appreciate this interconnection is useful in helping her to slow down and understand what is triggering her feelings

In support of a pivot from caretaker to coach, it is helpful for Claire to ask herself, "What would a coach do?" and to remember what a coaching role entails. As a coach, you step back from "doing for" and choose a different response to your young adult. You move to the passenger seat, and let your child be the driver. For Claire, and for

---

> ### EXHIBIT 2.4. Emotion Regulation Skills
>
> - Notice you are experiencing an emotion; note physiological changes in your body.
> - Sit with the emotion and label the emotion.
> - Take a breath and think about possible triggers for that particular emotion.
> - Accept your emotion without judgment.
> - Identify what you would like the other person to know.
> - Picture how you would like to come across to the other person.
> - Choose a response that will accurately communicate your feelings and your message.

---

many of us, this is a difficult shift. Once we are able to make this pivot to coach, we can engage in autonomy support with our young adult.

Set and Maintain Your Own Personal Boundaries

Much like physical boundaries (e.g., walls, fences), emotional boundaries give us a clear sense of where we end and another person begins, what is ours and what is theirs. When we have healthy boundaries, we can relate better to others and not get caught up in their storm. Likewise, the chaos we feel does not spill over onto them.

Let's look at the concept of boundaries from a continuum perspective. At one end of the continuum, we find a person with weak or nonexistent boundaries. This individual has no clear sense of themselves as a distinct being, and other people direct the course of their life. A parent with weak boundaries (see Figure 2.1, left) has little ability to make effective decisions for themselves and is likely to cave in to the demands of others including their young adult.

At the other end of the continuum is a person with such rigid boundaries that nothing much can get through (see Figure 2.1, right).

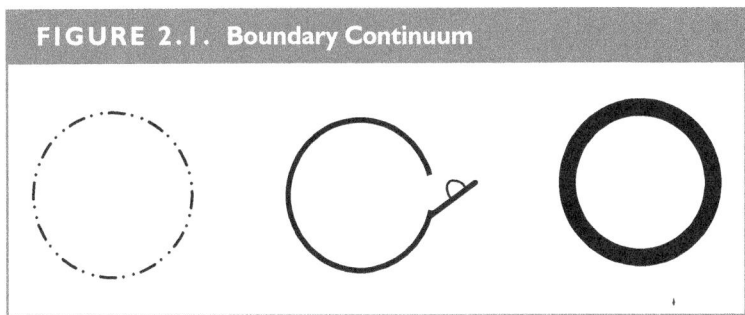

FIGURE 2.1. Boundary Continuum

Such a person has a narrow sense of self that is strongly resistant to input from others or shifts in circumstances. They are disconnected from others and quite often are unwilling to see things from a different perspective. Their ability to listen to others and adapt to changing situations is markedly impaired.

In the middle of the continuum is the person with relatively healthy boundaries—that is, they have a clear sense of themselves as a distinct being, and their boundaries are open to let others in when they so choose (see Figure 2.1, center). Healthy boundaries are different from weak or rigid ones in that they are firm yet will open and/or expand when you choose to open them to other people or new ideas. Healthy boundaries "breathe" with you as you go about your life, allowing you to adapt and adjust to the needs of the situation. You will note the opening on the circle that allows the person to open and expand the boundary when they deem it appropriate to let in new information. This includes being willing to listen to the ideas of and advice from others.

Returning to Claire, let's imagine she has weak boundaries; she can't make a decision, and so she watches Anne continue to reject any help with accommodations. Claire wrings her hands and feels helpless. On the other hand, if Claire has rigid boundaries, she may believe that the problem is Anne's to solve and step away or go on the offensive and dictate to Anne what she should do. Either way, there is little flexibility.

Claire's ability to set and maintain healthy boundaries will allow her to make appropriate decisions regarding her own actions with her daughter. Rather than give in to helplessness and leave Anne floundering, she will listen to input from her husband and not feel the need to go it alone in deciding how to handle the situation. She will also be flexible in how she interacts with Anne and adjust her approach as the situation evolves.

Support Autonomy

The skill of providing autonomy support can add significantly to the role of coach. Much of the literature on parental autonomy support is aimed at parents of children and teens; however, it has a lot to offer parents of emerging adults as well. It's important to remember the development of autonomy is essential to the process of emerging adulthood. Therefore, it makes sense that a parenting style supportive of autonomy would be highly effective with emerging adults. Autonomy supportive parenting is often contrasted with controlling parenting—where parents ignore the perspective of their young adult and instead manipulate them into carrying out the parents' expectations. Controlling parents threaten to take away privileges or to ground their adult child; they offer little or no empathy and little privacy, and they insert themselves into virtually every aspect of their young adult's life. This is all done with the aim of making sure their expectations for their adult child are met. Autonomy-supportive parents, on the other hand, encourage their emerging adult to be independent, and they impart confidence in their young adult's ability to solve problems and to make decisions (Kouros et al., 2017). Parents using autonomy support make every effort to listen to the thoughts and feelings of their young adult even during times of disagreement or conflict; they express their own emotions and share their rationale for their decisions. There is a relationship between autonomy support and autonomous motivation: Young adults choosing goals that, to them, are personally meaningful. An autonomy-supportive environment leads to increases in autonomous motivation and vice versa, with both resulting in positive emotion for emerging adults (Levine et al., 2021).

A recent *New York Times* article told the story of a special-education teacher who was diligently working to manage a classroom full of highly agitated students. When the author of the article asked the teacher to identify what works with students who are overwhelmed and upset, the teacher responded saying she relies on the use of one question: "Do you want to be helped, heard, or hugged?" (Dunn, 2023, para. 3). What a simple yet amazing question! It offers the student—or in your case, your young adult—a choice that affords them some control, while at the same time provides you, the parent, with an intervention that will meet your young adult's needs.

To better understand autonomy-supportive behavior, it might be helpful to take a look at the types of behavior that are not reflective of autonomy support. Let's imagine the following exchange between a parent and their emerging adult:

> *Emerging adult:* I'm thinking about taking next semester off to work and figure out what major I might like.
>
> *Parent:* What?! What are you thinking? This is not what we planned. All the money we spent will be wasted, and chances are good you won't go back! Forget it, you can't quit.

Here's another example:

> *Emerging adult:* Guess what? I've made a big decision; I'm going to join the Marines after I graduate from high school.
>
> *Parent:* Where in the world did that come from? Who planted this crazy idea in your head? I thought you were planning on taking a few weeks off and then looking for a job in sales. Absolutely not.

Does either of these sound like a reaction you might have to your emerging adult announcing they want to take a break from school or join the military? It certainly can catch you, or any parent, off guard. Your natural inclination might be to refuse to listen to such talk. You don't want them to quit school. At the same time, you are uncertain about how to proceed. Engaging your autonomy support skills will be necessary to resolve the situation in such a way that both you and your adult child feel understood and heard. In addition, your ability to show support for their decisions is a key factor in the process. This is difficult when their decisions seem fly-by-night and whimsical.

Now let's replay these same two situations but with autonomy-supportive behavior.

> *Emerging adult:* I'm thinking about taking next semester off to work and figure out what major I might like.
>
> *Parent:* (*Takes a breath and considers what they are feeling. They notice they are feeling shock and some anger after being caught off guard. They then begin to*

calm down). To be honest with you, this is very upsetting to me. I never expected this; I feel like it's coming out of nowhere.

Now for the second situation:

Emerging adult: Guess what? I've made a big decision; I'm going to join the Marines after I graduate from high school.

Parent: (*Takes a deep breath, identifies the predominant feeling of fear, and relaxes.*) Did I hear you say you want to join the Marines? What's going on here? I have to be honest, I wasn't expecting this.

Emerging Adult: A recruiter came to our school and told us about all the options offered by the military. I thought they sounded cool, and if I want to attend school later, the military would pay for it. I know it will be hard at first, but the benefits are so good.

Parent: I guess that makes some sense, but I really don't know much about the military. I need to think about this. How would you feel about each of us gathering more information and then talking about what we found together?

Can you see the difference in the dialogues when autonomy support skills are used? The parent in each case is obviously thrown for a loop, but after taking a minute to breathe and calm themselves, they are better able to respond in a way that will keep communication with their young adult open.

Do Self-Care

Last, but certainly not least, is the importance of monitoring your own mental and physical well-being as you pivot to the role of coach. As your adult child's stress intensifies and their ability to function drops, so, too, might your distress impact your ability to function effectively as a parent. It is essential for you to engage in self-care activities that reduce your stress and allow you to think clearly and act wisely.

Self-care means you intentionally engage in activities that preserve and/or enhance your sense of well-being at all levels, including physical, emotional, spiritual, personal, and professional. Some models of self-care use the concept of a self-care wheel based on the work of Saakvitne and Pearlman (1996) and the Olga Phoenix Project (2013). The wheel lists many examples of self-care activities to address the various dimensions, including physical (take a nap, take a walk, eat healthy, etc.), emotional (watch reruns of your favorite sitcom, hang out with people you enjoy, etc.), spiritual (stop to take in a sunset or sunrise, meditate, be open to not knowing, etc.), professional (set healthy limits with clients and/or colleagues, take a break during the day, leave work at work, etc.), and personal (learn a new hobby, make time for friends, relax, etc.). We engage in different self-care activities based on the situation in which we find ourselves. No matter what role we are in, self-care is an essential practice for keeping us on a steady course with our young adult.

SUMMARY

In this chapter, we discussed what might be the most difficult pivot of the parenting experience—the pivot from the role of caretaker to the role of coach. Information regarding parenting in general was provided, along with a description of the new role of coach; specific skills needed to be an effective coach were discussed in detail. Our goal was for parents to gain a new perspective on their role as parents and to move forward with a sense of confidence. In the next chapter, we present vital information about symptoms of anxiety, depression, and other forms of distress. We describe how these symptoms may look in your emerging adult. We then proceed to talk in depth about "the dragons," also known as problematic behaviors that emerging adults often turn to in an effort to cope with the distressing psychological symptoms they are experiencing. Examples of such behaviors include substance misuse, unhealthy eating and exercise, internet misuse, and so on. We offer signs to look for should you suspect your young adult is engaging with the dragons.

POINTS TO POCKET

- It's a whole new world: We need different tools to parent our young adults.
- The easiest and most effective thing to do when you are feeling stress is to breathe deeply.
- Listening to your adult child is a full-on mind–body experience.
- Your words have power: Use them wisely.
- If you don't know what to say, take a beat and think about what might be helpful.

II

UPSIDE DOWN
AND INSIDE OUT

CHAPTER 3

RIDING THE DRAGONS: UNHEALTHY COPING IN YOUNG ADULTS

> *Fairy tales are more than true: Not because they tell us that dragons exist. But because they tell us that dragons can be beaten.*
>
> —Neil Gaiman, *Coraline*

In the previous chapter, we introduced you to some useful tools for your tote bag to help both you and your young adult on your journey through their emerging adult years. We began equipping you with coach tools, and as we continue, we will add more tools to your tote bag and show you how to use them in various situations. In this chapter, we venture into the realm of the "dragons," which appear as forms of substance misuse, unhealthy eating, internet misuse, and risky and impulsive behaviors like sexual acting out and reckless driving. For the purposes of this book, the dragons we include here rear up as unhealthy coping mechanisms when emerging adults experience anxiety, depression, and other forms of psychological distress (see Figure 3.1).

Many of us can relate to the idea of having a stressful and chaotic day at work and coming home to a cup of tea, a glass of wine, or that leftover piece of yummy chocolate cake waiting on the kitchen counter to help us calm down and relax. Likewise, the dragons help young adults distract from or escape negative emotions. We view these unhealthy behaviors on a continuum with use on one end, misuse in the middle, and addiction on the other end. Our focus in this chapter is not on what clinicians define as psychological disorders (substance use disorders, eating disorders, internet

---

FIGURE 3.1. Dragon Spiral

anxiety, depression, & distress ⟶ DRAGONS ⟶
more anxiety, depression, & distress

---

addiction, etc.) but rather those patterns of use that could fall in the middle range of what we term *misuse*. We define misuse as a young adult engaging with the behavior or substance to an extent or with such frequency that it may begin to interfere with their ability to handle daily tasks and responsibilities. This corresponds to what we said previously about distress and functionality: The young adult is moderately high on the distress meter and somewhat low on the functioning meter. Such behavior may also start to impact important relationships.

Whether your adult child is living at home or away, your journey as a parent is a challenging one. From your perspective as a parent, it can be difficult to determine where your adult child's behavior falls on this continuum. Is their behavior indicative of misuse or a sign of something more serious? Once again, the answer here is complicated. Put on your coach hat and read on.

ANXIETY REARS ITS HEAD

Let's return to the story of Jessie and her mother, Rachel, whom you met in the Introduction. Here is Rachel talking about Jessie:

> Shortly after starting her new job Jessie had a panic attack. This was not the first time she had anxiety issues. Several times in high school she had what she called "episodes" where she would get very anxious, her heart would race, and she'd begin to gulp for air. During those times, I could usually talk her down from the episode, calming her and helping her recenter

and breathe. I tried to get Jessie to see someone at the clinic in town to help her deal with the anxiety.

Jessie adamantly refused. "They're all your friends and coworkers. Why would I talk to any of them? They've been to our house for cookouts and stuff. Holy crap, Mom! No way!"

The symptoms of panic attacks, like those Jessie experienced, can be frightening. These episodes can be random or can occur in response to specific triggers. Ironically, the apprehension about the possibility of having another panic attack in the future can contribute to the likelihood of this happening. Most adults may experience one or two of these panic attacks in their lifetime. However, a small percentage of these adults have recurrent and severe attacks that may warrant a clinical diagnosis. And as is true for Jessie, these attacks often occur in combination with other symptoms of anxiety, such as worry, difficulty concentrating, and avoidance of people or places, as well as depression.

Although Jessie's symptoms were obvious to her mom, many times symptoms of anxiety and depression are not so easily detectable, especially if your adult child is not residing at home. Rachel is concerned, and possibly confused about what these symptoms mean for her daughter. Like many parents, Rachel may wonder if Jessie's anxiety is a temporary reaction to the stress that normally accompanies the stage of emerging adulthood or the beginning of a more serious mental health disorder. These fears can be compounded by the realization that many serious mental health disorders develop for the first time during this developmental stage. It is no wonder that parents worry and fear the worst. As you will learn in the next chapter, clarity about what Jessie's symptoms mean often entails a comprehensive evaluation by mental health providers. While the evaluation can be complex, the key to understanding and differentiating between normal growing pains and something more severe is determining the degree to which the symptoms cause your child distress or interfere with their ability to function in school, work, and interpersonal relationships.

Rachel is clearly concerned for her daughter. When faced with Jessie's reluctance to engage in mental health treatment, Rachel's stress level hit the roof. In the past, whenever concerns arose about Jessie's physical and mental health, Rachel sought help for her daughter and was an active part of the decision-making process regarding treatment. Now that Jessie is over 18, the rules change. We discuss the health care implications of your adult child becoming a legal adult in Chapter 6. For right now, it would help Rachel to remember to use one of her breathing techniques as she uses the skills of the coach role to help Jessie.

While Rachel was aware of Jessie's problem and encouraged her to seek professional help, this is not always possible. In many instances adult children are gone from the home and contact with parents is limited. In other instances, signs and symptoms are not always easy for parents to recognize. For example, depressive symptoms are sometimes not obvious; they can be exhibited in emerging adults as frequent complaints about bodily aches and pains including headaches and digestive issues. Some young adults, like adolescents, are more apt to exhibit irritability instead of sadness. Depression can be experienced as a sense of numbness or emptiness as well as sadness. Apathy is common and may appear even when your adult children are participating in activities previously enjoyed. Your adult child may be argumentative and engage in acting-out behavior, creating unnecessary conflict. Young adults may also come across as pessimistic and sarcastic. Your emerging adult may seem unmotivated and inattentive to simple tasks such as showering, doing the laundry, and preparing food. Because these behaviors are developmentally typical for this age group, you may not easily recognize them as signs of depression or anxiety. The emerging adults who lack energy or motivation—potential signs of depression—may simply sleep their way through the morning or make excuses for not getting to work or school on time: "My friends all sleep till one in the afternoon." As a parent, you may write this off to your adult child just being lazy.

Like Jessie, young adults report more anxiety and depression than any other age group (Goodwin et al., 2020; Villarroel & Terlizzi, 2020). These feelings may be temporary and can be associated with both positive events (e.g., a job promotion, a new romantic relationship) and negative events (e.g., job loss, injury/illness, relationship breakup). As you know, the stage of emerging adulthood is fraught with heightened stress, anxiety, and worry. Hence, the need to make decisions, especially those with lifelong implications, results in increased pressure, making such decisions even more difficult. Wearing that coach hat, you can listen intently and with empathy to your young adult, using open-ended questions to get them to talk about what they are experiencing. Even though what they tell you may trigger strong feelings, you will be best served by regulating your emotional responses and respecting their autonomy by not overreacting or trying to make their decisions for them. Keep these skills in mind as we now meet the dragons.

 ## ENTER THE DRAGONS

Stop for a minute. Take a deep breath; you may find yourself personalizing some of the information we present here and questioning your own behavior regarding your relationship with one or more of the dragons. This may raise your own level of distress. Get your tote bag ready and keep the continuum in mind as we enter the realm of the dragons. A major requirement for any athletic coach is having an in-depth knowledge of the sport they are coaching. You may want to brew yourself a cup of coffee or hot tea as you settle in and read some important information about the dragons. Keep in mind that the dragons serve an important purpose: They provide a distraction for your young adult from the pressure and stress associated with this stage of life.

Substance Misuse in Young Adults

Remember that substance misuse is not the same as addiction. Misuse in this book refers to use of alcohol and drugs in a quantity and with a frequency beyond experimentation or social use. This misuse can result in increased risk for physical and psychological harm as well as family, social, academic, occupational, and financial problems. It is important to stress that even a single episode of drug or alcohol misuse can lead to severe or even fatal outcomes.

Let's hear from Rachel as she recounts Jessie's next panic attack.

This time, Jessie was alone in her apartment when the attack overcame her. She called me at work, barely able to get words out to tell me what was happening. I was in the middle of a run to the hospital and couldn't get to Jessie for several hours. I called her brother Jared who was just getting home from soccer practice and asked him to go check on Jessie. By the time I got to Jessie's apartment, my son and daughter were sitting on the couch grinning and laughing foolishly. They had each consumed a cannabis gummy and were feeling no pain. I stared at them for a moment, then slowly sank into a chair. What was happening? My kids didn't do drugs. Did they? And where did they get them if they did?

Sure, I smoked pot occasionally when I was younger, but nothing more. My husband had been a straight arrow, and we raised our children to steer clear of drugs. I used to have a beer or a glass of wine with him at dinner time, but nothing else. After all I see in the ER at work, I wanted no part of any of the street drugs so many young people were getting their hands on. And I most certainly did not want my kids having access to any of it. I wish for the umpteenth time that my husband was alive to help me. I am scared to death and feel so alone in this. I have no idea what to say to my daughter. I freeze in place.

On several fronts, Jessie and Jared's use of marijuana is not surprising. The stages of adolescence and emerging adulthood are normally associated with experimentation, risk-taking, and impulsivity. When this is combined with greater freedom and less control, it is not surprising that Jessie discovers pot gives her some temporary relief and maybe even serves as a distraction from her anxiety. When faced with unpleasant or uncomfortable emotions and stress, many adults engage in the use of substances as a form of self-medication. Most adults, and especially young adults, look for quick fixes. These quick fixes can also be found in other behaviors such as misuse of alcohol and other drugs, unhealthy eating and exercising, internet misuse, high-risk sexual behaviors, and other reckless behavior. Such behaviors can function as a temporary escape or a way of self-medicating. As young adults begin to build a more independent life, their eating patterns, internet use, substance use, and sexual activity are likely not as obvious to you as they once were. When this is combined with the pressure in some social contexts, such as college life, to consume alcohol, pot, and other drugs, the connection between your adult child's emotional distress and problematic coping behaviors is more firmly established. A toxic stew begins to boil when the misuse of substances and other dragons are coupled with anxiety, depression, and other emotional distress. In fact, it is common among young adults for these symptoms to commingle and worsen over time.

In our experience, many parents tend to either overreact or underreact in situations like this. For example, some parents might let loose a barrage of accusations and blow the situation out of proportion. On the other end of the continuum, some parents may laugh it off (e.g., "it's only weed, it's not heroin") or ask to join the party. In either case, the over- or underreaction likely diverts attention away from addressing the underlying distress the emerging adult feels. It may actually fuel continued use on the part of the young adult. In Rachel's case, she alludes to the fact that she feels frozen, and perhaps this opens up a possible middle ground that allows her to pause and consider how to respond. However, it is important to stress that some people do remain frozen.

Instead, we encourage you to make a conscious decision to pause and consider how to respond as a coach in the situation. This is a great time to open your tote bag and pull out some tools (listening intently; using clear, deliberate communication; employing empathy; maintaining healthy boundaries; using emotion regulation and self-care; etc.) that are associated with the coaching role you learned about in Chapter 2. For example, simply breathing in and out reduces your stress or anxiety in the moment. This is a good time to consider when and how you might talk with your adult child about what you observed.

There are many reasons young adults misuse substances, including for exploration and experimentation, to gain social acceptance or avoid rejection, and to enhance athletic and academic performance. They also use substances as a way to cope with anxiety, depression, and the stress associated with daily life. This negative coping is the most damaging of these motivations (Gregg et al., 2014). However, the use of substances to cope with stress, to numb one's feelings, or to avoid and to alleviate unpleasant or noxious feelings is especially compelling for young adults. Unfortunately, even though young adults think these substances will lessen their anxiety, depression, and general distress, they actually make these feelings worse.

When emerging adults use increasingly larger quantities of substances over sustained periods of time and beyond social norms, they are at risk for developing more serious problems. The misuse of these substances is especially concerning due to its potential long-term consequences on brain health. The human brain is not fully developed until around age 25. This means your young adult's capacity to manage emotions, problem solve, and control impulses is not fully established. Substance use during this period acts to "prime" the brain and make young people more vulnerable to addiction (C. J. Jordan & Andersen, 2017).

Emerging adults misuse substances more than any other age group (National Institute on Drug Abuse & the National Institutes of Health, 2020). One form of substance misuse is binge drinking (four drinks in a row for women, five for men); this is the most common form of alcohol misuse in young adults with estimates ranging from 30% to 40% of the college population (Krieger et al., 2018). College students report more binge drinking than their non–college student counterparts (Arnett, 2015).

Research evidence suggests that cannabis misuse among emerging adults has also increased (Schulenberg et al., 2017). Much of this may be attributed to the fact that it has been legalized in many locations and is also prescribed for medical use. Although the public perception of risks associated with cannabis use may have shifted, when young adults are consistently using pot to cope with anxiety, depression, and other forms of emotional distress, they could be putting themselves in harm's way.

The misuse of opioids (e.g., oxycodone, hydrocodone) and stimulants (e.g., Adderall, Ritalin) by emerging adults, particularly those who are between 18 and 25, is the highest, relative to all other age groups in the United States (Hughes et al., 2016). Opioid misuse among young adults in the United States is an epidemic. Misuse of both these types of drugs poses risks for serious adverse outcomes including drug dependence and accidental overdose (Substance Abuse and Mental Health Services Administration, 2017). Negative mood states such as anxiety and depression are consistently associated with more severe nonmedical use of opioids (Bakhshaie et al., 2019). In contrast, stimulant misuse among young adults is most often prompted by a desire to enhance concentration and academic performance (Drazdowski, 2016).

We would be remiss if we didn't discuss the use of nicotine among emerging adults. Over the past few decades, the rates of cigarette smoking have declined, but the use of electronic cigarettes (e-cigarettes) among adolescents and young adults has grown in the United States (Glasser et al., 2019). E-cigarettes contain nicotine or tetrahydrocannabinol (THC), along with flavorings and other additives that create a vapor that users inhale. In contrast to older adults, emerging adults are not necessarily attracted to e-cigarettes because they want to quit smoking (Kinouani et al., 2020). Young adults are motivated by curiosity and the flavoring or taste of e-cigarettes, clever packaging and promotion, or because they perceive these to be less harmful compared with other tobacco products. Although emerging adults are initially simply curious about e-cigarettes, their continued use is often motivated by the need to manage stress and anxiety (Holt et al., 2024). E-cigarette misuse in young adults is associated with harmful consequences including lung damage, nicotine addiction, and future cigarette and other substance use (Gupta & Kalagher, 2021).

If this sets off alarm bells for you right now and you are experiencing a flood of thoughts and feelings, you are not alone. As a parent, your reactions may be influenced by the nature of the substance your young adult is misusing and the social stigma associated with it. For example, parents may be far less upset upon discovering their adult child's binge-drinking episode than they would be to learn that their adult child has tried oxycodone for recreational purposes. Remember to use those breathing techniques when you need them, coach!

As clinicians we have observed that parents often feel guilty and worry that their own or another family member's substance misuse may have contributed to their young adult's problems with substances. Parents may minimize their adult child's use of substances to mask their own misuse. They may see their adult children's use of alcohol as age-appropriate and be dismissive, even when obvious warning signs of misuse are present. In these cases, it is important for parents to learn how to forgive themselves for their past mistakes. In Chapter 9, we address these issues in more depth and provide you with some tools to manage these issues more effectively. Dealing with your adult child's substance misuse can also awaken childhood memories of growing up in alcoholic or drug-abusing families. In these situations, it is often helpful for parents to have their own safe space either with a trusted friend, therapist, or confidant to talk through these complex dynamics.

Uncertainties about the nature and extent of your adult child's substance misuse and its effects can also complicate decisions about whether and how to talk with them about their substance use. Some parents may adopt a "don't ask, don't tell" policy about the use of alcohol and marijuana because they don't think these substances can be particularly harmful. As a parent, you may avoid confronting your adult child for fear of alienating them or worry that any intervention in their life would be counterproductive to their need for autonomy. Sometimes you are just plain anxious about the prospect of doing so.

Whether your general tendency as a parent is to approach or avoid conflict, you may find yourself paralyzed by fear, either by the fear of having no idea what to do or the fear of doing the wrong thing. Whatever your particular situation, we encourage parents to communicate constructively with their adult children. However, it is important that parents prepare for these difficult conversations and have their tote bags with coaching tools readily available.

Your young adult must feel as though they are in an emotionally safe space before anything more can happen. They need to know that they won't be attacked or belittled by mom or dad, or both. For example, imagine that Rachel turned to Jessie and said, "Where's your judgment? How could you suddenly think it was okay for you to start using pot? And how could you ever think it was okay to involve Jared?" This is an attack, not a question; Jessie is likely to go on the defensive, and communication shuts down.

For Rachel, it will be important to stage a conversation with Jessie about her marijuana use when they are both in a relaxed mode, at a time when interruptions are not likely to occur in a context where they will not be overheard by others. For example, taking a drive together or taking a walk side-by-side with your adult child may minimize possible emotional intensity that comes through direct eye contact and is an effective way to down-regulate any feelings of stress or anger on both sides. As coach, a parent needs to listen intently without judging or critiquing. Open-ended statements would also serve you well. Let's return to Rachel's dialogue with Jessie: "Tell me more about what happened" or "Help me to understand what was going on when Jared got involved." Here, you are seeking first to understand what is going on with your young adult before you seek to be understood yourself.

Even though you might not agree with your adult child's coping strategy, they need to know you have their back. Once they know it is safe, they will be in a better place to tell you what's going on and talk about what they are feeling. It is important to underscore the point that the behavior—in this case, their substance misuse—is signaling something, perhaps the presence of an underlying mental health issue. And that something needs to be named. Breaking news: This is not easy to do. One of the challenges of doing this is separating your adult child's behavior from your adult child as well as seeing them as separate from you. They are not an extension of you, and they are not defined by their behavior.

Exploring your young adult's motivations for using substances is important. In Jessie's case, it is likely that pot use provided temporary relief from her anxiety. Rachel might want to use open-ended questions to explore alternative ways Jessie could cope with her anxiety. It is important to remember that in the coaching role, the parent is not directing their young adult to stop using pot or advising them in other ways. The parent is, however, asking them to engage in active problem-solving.

Unhealthy Eating and Exercise

Young adults frequently have an unhealthy relationship with food (e.g., overeating, using food to soothe emotions, feeling depressed and guilty after eating, counting calories, labeling good and bad foods). Given the cultural emphasis on physical appearance and the many challenges of emerging adulthood, it is not surprising that young adults, women in particular, explore a number of unhealthy eating and weight-control behaviors. Research findings show about one quarter of emerging adults engage in unhealthy weight-control behaviors (Gonidakis et al., 2018).

Healthy exercise offers physical, emotional, and social benefits for young adults and is highly recommended. Unfortunately, some emerging adults tend to overexercise. Overexercise is characterized by excessive and obsessive exercise and serves as a compensatory behavior when too many calories have been consumed. Overexercise often accompanies an unhealthy relationship with food. Our purpose here is to discuss unhealthy eating, not eating disorders, as a response to anxiety, depression, and other forms of emotional distress for some young adults. Emerging adults may engage in unhealthy eating behaviors to cope with stress and uncomfortable emotions. Again, we turn to the continuum to aid you in gaining a better understanding of your young adult's relationship with food. We begin with healthy eating on one end, unhealthy eating in the middle, and disordered eating on the other end. The latter refers to patterns of eating that are consistent with an eating disorder diagnosis.

A young adult who demonstrates healthy eating consumes not only a variety of foods, but also an adequate amount of food; they eat regularly without guilt, and they enjoy treats or "fun" foods. Those adult children who exhibit unhealthy eating tend to undereat, overeat, or both; they avoid what they might term "bad" or "forbidden" foods, they engage in yo-yo dieting, and they often overexercise. On the far right of the continuum are those emerging adults who demonstrate disordered eating. Disordered eating can range from severe restriction leading to significant weight loss to binge eating accompanied by vomiting, laxative use, strict rules around eating, and rigid and excessive exercise. Your adult child's relationship with food could fall anywhere along the continuum, and it is subject to change based on their life circumstances.

If you should notice your emerging adult engaging in an unhealthy relationship with food, it is important to note that not all unhealthy eating is aimed at weight loss or a change in body image. For some young adults, their behaviors with food might offer them a sense of control over their bodies. This is particularly true of those emerging adults who experienced trauma in the form of physical or emotional abuse as well as those who may have had some form of medical procedure when they were younger. Some adult children practice an unhealthy relationship with food in an attempt to rebel or assert themselves against parental expectations they believe to be unrealistically high or unreasonable. These young adults likely experience their parents as highly controlling over many aspects of their lives.

Perhaps a more common motivation for the development of unhealthy eating behaviors is as a means of managing negative emotions, particularly anger. This is especially true for females, given the unfavorable view of expressed anger from women and girls in mainstream society. Their goal is to stuff their uncomfortable feelings with food rather than express their emotions verbally and directly.

If you do suspect your adult child is engaging in an unhealthy relationship with food, you are likely feeling overwhelmed, frightened, and uncertain how to proceed. Before sitting down with your young adult, it might be helpful for you to reflect on your own relationship with food, both current and past. It is also important to understand that your words and what you model as a parent have power and that teasing or offhand remarks (e.g., "hey, butter-butt," "nice muffin-top") even from childhood can have long-standing, negative effects. It's so easy to communicate messages through our own behavior to our children, teens, or young adults without even realizing it. Examples include skipping meals, reading the calories on packages while shopping, weighing yourself frequently, and making comments about your weight or clothing size. If you suspect this may have occurred, keep it in mind as you plan a dialogue with your emerging adult. The goal is not for you to feel blame but rather to use your insight as you try to understand your young adult's relationship with food.

The idea of initiating a dialogue with your young adult is likely creating some stress for you. Take a deep breath, pick up your tote bag, and take a look at the effective communication skills you learned in Chapter 2. We recommend you begin by inviting your adult child to sit down for a discussion with you regarding some concerns you would like to share. Take the time to identify carefully the behaviors you have been observing, then share or describe your feelings about the behaviors. Don't vent! Remember to use "I" rather than "you" statements. Give your emerging adult some time to respond. Keep in mind, your young adult may respond with denial or anger. Once they start talking, even if they are angry, listen and continue to listen for as long as they wish to talk. Be patient and keep your focus on them. When you do respond, respond with empathy and support. Chances are you may feel like crying or screaming; you can process your own emotions later. Right now, your focus is your young adult and your message is one of love and ongoing support.

When discussing unhealthy eating behaviors with your adult child, there are a few things it's best to avoid. The first is commenting on their weight or any aspect of their appearance. Such comments could serve to reinforce the idea that weight or appearance are all that matter. We also encourage you to refrain from making comments about your own weight or that of other people because such comments could have the same effect. Your adult child needs to switch their focus to who they are on the inside. The second is "you" statements that imply blame. Chances are your young adult lacks a solid sense of self and may perceive themselves as having little value. Suggesting blame in any way will only distance your adult child and maybe even result in a decision to continue their unhealthy behaviors with food.

If you choose to communicate your own thoughts and feelings to your emerging adult, make sure you use "I" statements. For example, "I feel concerned and anxious when you refer to yourself as fat" as opposed to "I think you are obsessed with your weight." And the third is offering solutions. Unhealthy eating patterns can take time to emerge, and they are often difficult to unravel. There is no easy solution for unhealthy eating, and the suggestion of one might imply your young adult is doing something wrong. Patience here is imperative! Remember your goal is to begin a dialogue with your emerging adult; it is not to arrive at a solution.

Internet Misuse

There are many reasons your adult child logs onto the internet. Emerging adults use their smartphones, tablets, and computers as a means of browsing for information, for entertainment, to connect socially with others, and alleviate their boredom. Internet activities such as online shopping, gaming, gambling, and pornography are easily accessible and affordable and include stimulating visual and interactive content. The internet affords young adults the capacity to experience and express themselves with fewer inhibitions while remaining anonymous to a certain degree.

Young adults who are just starting college and are without a social support network may initially come to rely on social media as a way of filling this void. During the COVID-19 pandemic, forced isolation, boredom, and reliance on online learning platforms were especially conducive to the heightened use of social media.

As with other dragons, we propose that internet use behavior falls on a continuum, with use on one end and on the other end, internet addiction. By *internet addiction*, we are referring to the uncontrollable need to spend more and more time on the computer, to the point that aspects of life (e.g., social relationships, academics, personal hygiene) are ignored. *Internet misuse* refers to involvement in internet activity to such an extent that it may negatively impact daily life, including school- and job-related responsibilities, family relationships, and friendships, and may contribute to low mood. The sedentary aspect of internet misuse may be problematic from a health perspective and may lead to weight issues, blurred vision, neuromuscular complaints, and sleep deprivation. Internet addiction is not currently recognized in the current *Diagnostic and Statistical Manual of Mental Disorders* (5th ed., text rev.; American Psychiatric Association, 2022) as a clinical disorder, as it is in some countries (e.g., China, Korea, Taiwan). In real life, defining the point at which your young adult crosses the line from general internet use to internet misuse is somewhat murky.

Let's hear from Pete about Ian's internet use.

I got increasingly concerned as Ian continued to show no signs of shutting down his computers or looking for work. He was online every single time I went down to his room, even at 1 in the morning. I decided to take action and confronted him when he "came up for air" and food one day, 2 weeks after he got home.

"Ian," I said, "Take a seat with that sandwich. We need to talk."

Ian stuffed his mouth and reached for a soda from the fridge before sitting at the island in our kitchen. "What do you want to talk about?" he asked between bites.

I responded, "Well, first, your summer job, and second, the fact that you don't seem to be connecting with me or your friends this summer. Jeff and Mason have been calling, and you seem to be brushing them off. I'm concerned about you. I don't know what's going on."

Ian rolled his eyes, took another big bite and finished his sandwich. "Dad, I'm okay, alright? Don't worry about me."

"Too late, son," I responded. "I'm already there. What's going on?"

"Nothing."

"Blue sheets, Ian." (I had taken to saying this rather than the other meaning for B.S. when Ian was younger, to try to keep profanity to a minimum in our little family).

Ian smiled at this. "It was a tough semester, okay, Dad? I need to unwind a bit before I go out and look for work."

"It's been 2 weeks, Ian. I think it's time you got moving."

"I need more time."

"And I need to see some progress. I don't want to cut your cable off, or take the computers away, but I may not have a choice."

I saw the panicked look on Ian's face, and thought this might get him off his butt and moving. However, I was also beginning to suspect that the internet use was serving as something beyond simply whiling away the days. My mind started spinning in several directions as I contemplated the horrors my friends talked about with their adult kids and the internet and what I read about in the paper. I needed to figure out what was going on fast, for both Ian's sake and my own peace of mind.

Emerging adults are often motivated to engage in internet misuse to escape negative emotions or distract from stress. Ironically, feelings of anxiety, depression, and emotional distress can follow from the use of this technology. A vicious cycle can start when young adults begin spending time online for a temporary escape from negative feelings and thoughts and, in turn, negative consequences can exacerbate the emotional distress your young adult may already be experiencing and result in a further erosion of quality of life. If Pete is suspecting something else is going on with Ian, it is important to approach his son honestly with his concern and listen with empathy to what he says.

Rather than responding to the situation with directives and threats to pull the plug on the computers as a caretaker might do, in his coach role, Pete needs first to recognize that his thoughts and fears about what might be going on are irrational on some level (after all, it is unlikely that Ian is gambling away his college fund). Pete also needs to find out the facts concerning Ian's behaviors thus far before he goes on the offensive. It would be helpful for Pete to walk back the threat of cutting off all internet use and instead focus on what his son said about it being a rough semester. If this is done in a calm, nonjudgmental manner, Ian is more likely to open up and talk about what was rough rather than needing to defend himself.

Pete tries again the following week.

I approached Ian in a gentle manner when he seemed relaxed and said, "Ian, I'm getting really concerned about you spending so much time on your computer and phone. I've noticed that you sit for hours at a time in front of the screen, and you are up really late at night. You said you had a tough semester. I'd really like to hear more."

At this point I could see Ian tense up. I waited, then asked in a quiet voice, "I'd like to hear about it, son."

Ian's shoulders slumped, and he looked at me. "I'm worried I can't make it at school. Everyone seems so much smarter than me. I busted my tail for the grades I got. It was really hard. My friends all say it was so easy for them. Well, it wasn't for me. I don't know if I even want to go back, Dad."

I took a beat and some deep breaths. This was not what I expected to hear. Ian had always done well in school. I finally said, "It must have been a struggle for you. Tell me more about it."

Ian sighed heavily. "It was like when I was in fourth grade and Mrs. Casey was teaching us to multiply fractions. I just couldn't figure out how to do that, and I felt so dumb."

"I remember you coming home from school and crying while you tried to do the homework," I said.

"Well, it's that same feeling, but in every class. It's like they're speaking a foreign language!"

I knew this was not the time to challenge the "every class" statement, so instead I offered support and said, "I get that. I can see now that being online all day is a great way to block out all the stress about not being able to make it."

Ian looked at me and heaved a sigh. "Yeah, I'm good at it and that's exactly why I do it, Dad. When I'm online gaming or scrolling through TikTok I don't have to think about that stuff."

Pete gained some valuable information regarding his son and how the internet was helping him cope. By encouraging Ian to talk rather than bombarding him with questions, he was able to move the conversation along without criticism or having Ian shut down. Clear, deliberate communication is crucial in helping you understand what your young adult is experiencing. When you have your own emotions under control, you can engage with your young adult without judging and also support their autonomy. These skills are all part of the coach role.

Young adults are especially susceptible to experiencing anxiety generated from the "fear of missing out" (FOMO; Deleuze et al., 2019; Li et al., 2015; Rasmussen et al., 2020). The ability through means of technology to discover what one is actually "missing" via smartphone notifications actually increases the fight-or-flight response described in Chapter 2. Once alerted, emerging adults reach for their cell phones on average, 82 times per day (Deloitte, 2016).

According to Spitzer et al. (2023), 90% of young adults reported using social network sites (TikTok, Instagram, Snapchat, Facebook, etc.) with as many as 84% reporting daily use of social media. Many believe the use of social media has displaced face-to-face communication for many young adults. Unfortunately, much of the young adult's time spent on social media involves making comparisons between themselves and their online connections. Young adults tend to favor Instagram because it offers a filtering function that allows young adults to create the most perfect images possible. Regrettably, these emerging adults frequently forget this filtering feature when making comparisons and may often wrongly perceive themselves as inferior or "less than." Researchers have found the more intensely young adults worry and experience themselves as inferior to their peers, the more likely they are to engage in self-harm behaviors and feel depressed (Hwang, 2019; Sherlock & Wagstaff, 2019; Spitzer et al., 2023).

As a parent you may be concerned about your adult child's attachment to their cell phone, tablet, laptop, or other electronic devices. The addictive nature of these activities coupled with the young adult's drive for excitement and experimentation can often lead to negative consequences down the road. You may secretly yearn for web content filtering software and internet blocker devices that you could use when your young adult was an adolescent. Unfortunately, these remedies are now considered an invasion of your adult child's much-coveted privacy. That being said, you might continue to wonder if your emerging adult is misusing the internet.

In so many instances, adult children are away from home and parents are simply not aware of their emerging adult's online activities. Young adults can "unfriend" or block their parents' access to their social networking sites. Rapid changes in technology and social media often contribute to the disconnect between parents and their emerging adults.

If you have the opportunity to observe your young adult directly, here are some signs and symptoms that indicate internet misuse: disruption in sleep patterns, physical discomforts (e.g., back or neck pain), forgetfulness, tardiness, less involvement in real-world relationships, absenteeism from work or classes, low grades or poor job performance, financial difficulties, irritable or depressed mood, and dishonesty regarding internet use. These signs are likely those seen with other dragons mentioned in this chapter.

Some parents may not perceive their adult child's internet use as a legitimate or desirable form of social interaction and may over-react to what they are seeing. In many cases, parents who grew up without the internet find excessive use of social media, gaming, and other internet activities more frightening than is the case with alcohol and drug misuse. It is also possible that parents might find themselves similarly wedded to their smartphones and other devices and there-fore downplay their adult child's use. These issues can complicate decisions about whether and how to talk with them about aspects of their internet use.

Let's imagine the following scenario. Your adult child is home from college during spring break and you are both enjoying a dinner out together. You note that your young adult spends significant stretches of time ignoring you because they are so absorbed in their phone—a phenomenon known as "phubbing" (a combination of "phone" and "snubbing"). Even when they are engaged in conversa-tion with you, they stop and check their cell phone every few min-utes. After a few rounds of phone checking, you find yourself feeling increasingly annoyed. However, you are hesitant to say something. As a parent, you think it may be too late to effect change in your young adult's use of technology. It is important to remember that if you would like to see some changes in your adult child's behavior, a good place to start might be to reflect on your own use of technol-ogy. For example, you might want to consider the fact that your children might really need your attention when you are busy looking at Facebook on your phone. It is our opinion that parents can and often do model behaviors for their children, no matter their ages. If the number of self-help books and advice columns on how to man-age your use of technology is any indication, finding a balance is a formidable challenge for adults of any age.

Modeling healthy internet use begins with actively considering your personal relationship with your own electronic devices. First, monitor the number of times you use your devices including phones, tablets, computers, and others. Ask yourself what emotions you feel before and after you use technology. It is quite possible that you may be using technology to cope or distract yourself from particular feelings and thoughts. Price (2018) recommended you use the acronym "WWW: What are you using technology for? Why now versus later? and What else can you be doing right now?" (p. 93). Several strategies for self-management are likely to aid you as a parent in modifying your own use and therefore better positioning yourself as a model for your adult child. See Exhibit 3.1.

 ## Other High-Risk and Reckless Behaviors

High-risk behaviors are defined as potentially dangerous, sensation-seeking actions where precautions that could be undertaken are not.

EXHIBIT 3.1. Strategies to Help You Get a Handle on Your Technology Use
• Turn off your notification function except for phone calls and calendar notifications. • Establish "no phone zones" (e.g., no phone at dinner table, bedroom, etc.). • Set "lock screen" function on your phone to remind you to go no further; place a rubber band around your phone to remind you to go no further. • Delete social media from your phone. • Take a digital sabbatical periodically. • Declutter your devices and delete old documents, emails, photographs, newsfeeds, and games.

These behaviors include reckless driving (e.g., drag racing, not stopping at traffic lights) and high-risk sexual behaviors (e.g., unprotected vaginal and anal sex, multiple sex partners) and are most prevalent during the stage of emerging adulthood (Willoughby et al., 2021). Let's stop for a moment and consider reckless driving, one of the dragons, from the perspective of Claire, Anne's mother.

> I was at work one day when out of the blue, my younger daughter, Sara, called in a panic.
>
> "Mom," she choked out between sobs, struggling for composure, "Anne . . . driving home from school . . . it was awful!"
>
> Sara took a breath before continuing. "I put my instruments and backpack on the back seat and climbed in beside Anne. She floored the gas pedal and took off. She continued to speed, then slammed on the brakes, then hit the gas again. I was so scared we were going to wreck. I begged Anne to slow down and be careful, but she didn't listen. She kept driving that way until we got home."
>
> I listened to Sara's recounting of the ordeal. I wasn't surprised Anne misdirected her frustration onto her driving. She would speed at times when she was frustrated or upset about something. I was surprised and angry, however, that she chose to put herself and her sister in harm's way. This was the first time to my knowledge that she drove this way with a passenger in the car.
>
> In a more composed manner Sara continued, "When I got out of the car, Anne sped off with my instruments and backpack still on the backseat. I yelled at her to stop and let me get my stuff, but she ignored me."
>
> I was too upset to remain at work, so I left to go home and deal with the situation. Anne arrived shortly after I did, and I took her aside to talk about her behavior and how she put herself and her sister in danger. I told her I expected more from her. She defended herself by saying she should not have to wait so long for her sister. She never really acknowledged

what she did or the impact of her behavior on Sara. Within a couple hours, she began acting like nothing had happened. This was her way of signaling that, as far as she was concerned, the conversation was over.

This behavior is apt to shake you, like Claire, to the core. When Claire relates the car incident to her husband, they are both concerned that Anne put herself and Sara in danger without considering the consequences. Experimentation, risk-taking, impulsivity, and emotionally driven decision-making are common characteristics of emerging adulthood, but they can result in serious injury, and even death (Mignault et al., 2022; Sawyer et al., 2018). This is not an easy reality for any parent to live with. These dragons can be overwhelming. Some of them may even remind you of your own struggles on the road to adulthood.

Claire and Stan decide that the first step would be for Claire to initiate a conversation with Anne. One thing Claire might do as coach in this situation is to first attend to regulating her own emotions. By calming herself through breathing exercises, she will be able to think more clearly and assess how and when to approach Anne. She will need to wait until she perceives Anne's distress is lower, and she seems able to listen to her mother. Claire can then sit down with her daughter and talk about her concern regarding the safety issues for both Anne and her sister in the driving incident. In doing this, Claire will need to listen and validate Anne's emotions, while gaining an understanding of what led to the behavior. Claire needs to stress her concern for her daughters' safety and well-being and use open-ended statements (e.g., "Help me to understand how you were feeling that day . . .") to encourage Anne to open up and explain what was going on with her. These coach skills will enable Claire to have a productive conversation with Anne and avoid blame or criticism.

Risky sexual practices are another dragon that can terrify you as a parent. As the Centers for Disease Control and Prevention (2016) reports, sexually transmitted infections (STIs) are on the rise among young adults. This increase could likely be attributed to high rates of unprotected sex and the use of dating apps. Dating apps (e.g., Tinder, Grindr) are popular among young adults in the United States; they are inexpensive, easy to use, and, as mobile apps, they can go anywhere. Young adults use dating apps to have fun, meet new people, and be social/chat with others (Sawyer et al., 2018). Frequent use of these apps is also linked to high-risk sexual behaviors, including unprotected vaginal and anal sex.

We see an example of this as Claire relates the following story about her daughter:

> Anne suddenly became preoccupied with her appearance, something she never bothered with too much. She also began surfing online dating apps and would tell me about various men she met.
>
> "What's a dating app?" I asked her, attempting a joke.
>
> She just scowled at me and stomped away. In truth, I was in shock! Anne never even liked social media and had no use for online apps before. Truth was, I do know that many young people use dating apps to hook up without incident. I have also heard stories in the media about young women who were tricked by men posing on these dating apps as someone they were not. I was concerned for her safety, and I talked with her about the need to exercise caution. She reacted angrily and stormed away.
>
> Anne also started having frequent casual sex with men she barely knew. She would tell me about these men to get a reaction. She defended her new behavior by telling me again and again that she felt good about herself and saw nothing wrong in what she was doing. I, on the other hand, was constantly worried about the potential consequences of her actions. I had no idea who this young woman was anymore. This is not how we raised her.

On the one hand, Claire was appalled at her daughter's seemingly promiscuous behavior. She had to stop, take a breath, and consider how different the attitudes toward women and their sexual behaviors were when she was Anne's age. Back then, young women were criticized and judged for being sexually active. They bore the brunt of society's double standard regarding sexual norms. On the other hand, Claire realized that women today have much more freedom to make their own decisions regarding their sexuality. She understands the reality of the current times, and yet she still worries about the impact of Anne's behavior on her physical and emotional well-being.

Claire was aware of these behaviors because her daughter was bragging about them. However, parents do not always know what their adult child is engaged in, especially if their young adult does not live at home. As with any of the high-risk behaviors, sometimes parents only find out because of the consequences—for example, if there is a car accident or their child is physically injured in some way or develops a medical condition as a result of the behavior.

High-risk sexual behaviors in young adults are often accompanied by alcohol misuse and can result in STIs and unplanned pregnancies. High rates of alcohol use on college campuses and, perhaps, changing expectations about casual dating and hookups, contribute to alarmingly high rates of sexual assault, otherwise termed "incapacitated rapes," where one partner is too intoxicated to consent or resist (Jaffe et al., 2023; Koss et al., 2022). Alcohol misuse can impair a young adult's ability to assess important cues about personal safety and may alter their ability to detect and correct misperceptions about intentions regarding sexual contact. Emerging adults who experience incapacitated rape can suffer a number of physical and mental health issues including depression and anxiety disorders, posttraumatic stress disorder, eating disorders, and others. These experiences can also contribute to the use of maladaptive coping

EXHIBIT 3.2. Calming Exercise: Gaze at a Color

- Focus on a color that you see in front of you (preferably your favorite color or one that relaxes you).
- Take a deep breath, as your eyes take in the hues of the color.
- Slowly shift your awareness to your breathing.
- While gazing at the color, inhale for 7 seconds and then slowly exhale.
- Immerse yourself in the color and let it calm your mind.

strategies such as substance misuse (e.g., binge drinking) to cope with the trauma. In addition, young adults who have experienced sexual assault are at greater risk for future revictimization.

You may feel confusion, guilt, or helplessness relative to your adult child's risky behaviors. Again, you are not alone in having these reactions. Dealing with your young adult's anxiety, depression, and associated high-risk behaviors may be particularly triggering for you if you experienced any or all of what are known as *adverse childhood events* (e.g., abuse, neglect, trauma, extreme family dysfunction, and your parent's substance abuse and/or mental health issues). Take a deep breath, and maybe try the calming exercise in Exhibit 3.2.

We invite you to continue reading to learn about tools to help you deal more effectively with your adult child and to lower your own stress level during these ongoing parenting challenges.

SUMMARY

As the parent of an emerging adult, you may not always be aware of when your young adult is anxious, depressed, or feeling otherwise distressed. These symptoms are often masked in this age group, and it may be challenging to differentiate between normative emerging adult behaviors and mood and anxiety symptoms. Likewise, as young adults begin to build a more independent life, their eating patterns, internet use, substance use, and sexual activities are likely not as obvious to you as they once were. It is probable, however, that your adult child's emotional distress and problematic behaviors are connected. A toxic stew can begin to boil when mood symptoms and these risky behaviors or dragons collide. In fact, it is common among young adults for these symptoms to commingle and intensify over time. At times parents may get sidetracked if substance misuse or risky sexual behaviors occur. In other words, this might become the focal point for parental concern and not the underlying anxiety, depression, and other emotional distress their adult child is experiencing. Using your coaching tools and the calming exercise we have offered so far will help you have more effective communication with your young adult and also keep your emotions in check and your stress from boiling over.

In Chapter 4, we provide parents with detailed information on the more serious mental health disorders to help parents get a better understanding of their young adult. Material related to self-harm and suicide is also presented. In Chapter 5, we discuss enhancing the coach role with advanced skills and provide parents with the tools necessary to communicate more effectively with their young adult. For those parents who suspect their adult child might be engaging with one or more of the dragons past the point of misuse or experience concerns about their own relationship with the dragon(s), we offer information regarding treatment access, provider options, and evidence-based treatment for both the dragons and serious mental health disorders.

POINTS TO POCKET

- Dragons are distractions: They help your young adult escape sadness, anxiety, loneliness, and other uncomfortable feelings.

- A coach needs to know the territory they are coaching: You need to understand the dragons that exist today that may not have been around when you were young.
- When you feel frustrated and helpless, remember: You can only control how you think and behave.
- It's hard to tell when the dragons cross the line into the danger zone. The best question is, does the dragon get in the way of your young adult's daily life? Dramatic changes in their behavior are red flags calling for a closer look.
- Understanding your own past and current dances with the dragons will help you better understand your young adult.
- Don't get sidetracked by the dragons; remember they may mask deeper psychological distress that needs to be addressed.

CHAPTER 4

THINGS FALL APART: SERIOUS MENTAL HEALTH ISSUES IN YOUNG ADULTS

Mental illness is so much more complicated than any pill that any mortal could invent.

—Elizabeth Wurtzel, *Prozac Nation*

Let's stop and take a breath. You've just stepped off the roller coaster ride with the dragons, and many parents find that to be a frightening and upsetting experience. Please know that you are not alone in this fear and remember to use the tools you already have in your tote bag to help you stay grounded. The chapter you are about to read contains information dealing with more serious forms of psychological distress—specifically, mental health disorders, which can be equally disturbing. To help you cope with such highly charged or unnerving material, we ask you to review some of the self-regulation (or self-soothing) tools we presented in Chapter 2 and introduce a critical new skill: Educate yourself! This is the first of several skills you will learn as you expand your mindset and skill repertoire to incorporate the role of *advanced coach*. This expansion of the coaching role is especially necessary when your young adult experiences more severe psychological distress and limited ability to function. In this chapter we concentrate on the skill of educating yourself. We will say more about the advanced coach role in the next chapter.

Remember the lightning bolt and spectacles are signals that the material you are about to read may be both highly charged and may take time for you to absorb. You might need to read the chapter more slowly to digest and make sense of it all. Take your time.

Are you ready? Okay, let's begin.

EDUCATE YOURSELF ABOUT SERIOUS MENTAL HEALTH DISORDERS

We turn our attention now to the presence of more serious mental health issues, which may transform the young adult you raised into someone you hardly recognize. Nearly everything about this person could change. Their lack of "rational" thinking or inability to attach consequences to their actions can push you to your limits. Educating yourself is the next essential skill in your development as a coach with your young adult. This skill is paramount to your understanding that mental illness may be driving your emerging adult's actions now. It is equally important to have some understanding about the illness itself to help you navigate the turbulence you are experiencing. When you are equipped with knowledge about what is going on with your young adult, you are better able to make effective decisions regarding what to do. The skill of educating yourself allows you to move forward with clearer vision, rather than stumble along not knowing what to do.

In this chapter, we present information about anxiety and mood disorders that are frequently seen in the young adult population. Keep in mind that only qualified mental health professionals can diagnose mental health disorders. We also discuss nonsuicidal self-injury, suicidal thoughts, and suicide attempts. For most parents, having knowledge about what their emerging adult is struggling with can help reduce the stress they are experiencing so that they can manage themselves and the situation more effectively. For now, we acknowledge once again that the information might provoke additional anxiety. Let's take another deep breath before reading further.

The onset and progression of mental health disorders can be gradual or abrupt, sporadic or ongoing. Typically, however, changes are slow and take months to develop. As changes in your adult child's mood, behavior, and perhaps also in their physical appearance become more obvious, chaos and conflict within the family can escalate. What begins as a discussion between you and your adult child may progress quickly into a shouting match. When parents share their concerns with their young adult, they can be met with a wall of anger, which can quickly intensify into verbal—and in some instances, physical—confrontations. Your sweet little child seems to have somehow morphed into an agitated and controlling young adult.

The stage of emerging adulthood is marked by continuing changes in the brain, body, and social environment. As such this is a highly stressful period for many young adults, with a considerable number experiencing symptoms that meet the diagnostic criteria for a mental health disorder. It is estimated that 75% of all mental illnesses begin during the stage of emerging adulthood, by age 24 (Kessler et al., 2005). The most common disorders in this stage and for young adults are anxiety and mood disorders.

Remember, for the purposes of our book, we use a continuum approach when talking about mental health disorders. We live in a world that likes to box things into neat categories such as good versus bad or yes versus no. Such categories suggest there is a clear judgment in one direction or the other. Experience teaches us, however, that the lines between such distinctions are far from clear. Each of us has our "off" days when we are just feeling down. These feelings can even vary throughout the day in terms of what we are doing and who we are with. In some situations, we may find our mood brightened by interactions with others, or alternatively our interactions may leave us down in the dumps. This feeling is fluid and not stuck in an on-versus-off mode. The feeling impacts our ability to function throughout the day, to a greater or lesser extent.

Chances are when we feel good, we move through the day with relative ease. However, when we're down, we are likely unfocused and lethargic. Likewise, your young adult's behaviors fall on a continuum in terms of their ability to function. And as we mentioned earlier, sleeping in on any given day is not uncommon for young adults, and few parents would bat an eye at that. However, sleeping in for 4 or 5 days in a row and missing work or classes may raise your level of concern.

Throughout this chapter, we use the phrase *more serious* to denote when the symptoms of depression, anxiety, or other emotional distress begin to affect a person's ability to function. In other words, they cross a line between what is considered typical in a given day for young adults and what reflects a clearer indication of impairment. As a parent, these symptoms can be quite disturbing. We provide a framework for you to understand what may be happening to your adult child and allow you to respond more effectively to their erratic behaviors.

At various points in this chapter, we refer to the universal question of "why is this happening to my child?" As clinicians, we are asked this question by countless parents. Unfortunately, there are no definitive answers. The more we know, the more we realize how much there is left to learn. The cause of any mental illness is likely the result of the interaction of multiple factors. The more we learn, the more we realize the complex or convoluted nature of virtually all forms of mental illness. For many years, researchers, providers, and the general public believed depression was primarily the result of abnormal levels of chemicals in the brain, specifically serotonin and norepinephrine, both neurotransmitters, also known as the body's chemical messengers. That belief has since been challenged (e.g., Moncrieff et al., 2023) and depression is now thought to be a result of the interaction of many factors, not just one. We understand how the desire for easy answers and quick fixes is so compelling right now, given the chaos and uncertainty surrounding us.

Likewise, mental health professionals need to understand symptoms such as anxiety, depression and other forms of emotional and behavioral distress in order to diagnose accurately and plan effective treatment. As you may know, the diagnostic manual used by mental health professionals, the fifth edition–text revision of the *Diagnostic and Statistical Manual of Mental Disorders* (*DSM-5-TR*; American Psychiatric Association, 2022), identifies criteria for each disorder including specific symptoms as well as their duration and severity. It is important to stress that medical doctors have access to blood tests, x-rays, and scans to help confirm a physical condition. However, at present, an accurate diagnosis of a mental disorder is considerably different. Such diagnoses rely on the self-report of the individual and the assessment skills of the mental health provider. A delay in the correct diagnosis only serves to increase the severity of the illness and therefore worsen its prognosis (i.e., the course of the illness moving forward). As we turn now to descriptions of the various disorders, remember that you are adding to your tote bag important knowledge that will help you manage your own stress as you deal with your young adult in distress.

ANXIETY IN YOUNG ADULTS

Emerging adults are at risk for developing anxiety disorders (Kessler et al., 2012) as these are the most commonly reported disorders among this age group. In our collective experience, generalized anxiety disorder, social anxiety, and panic disorder are frequently reported among young adults. For anxiety to become serious enough to cross the threshold to an anxiety disorder, it must be intense and uncontrollable. This means the symptoms impair one's ability to attend to daily life tasks for a duration of at least 6 months. If your young adult is dealing with more serious anxiety, they are likely experiencing continuous dread—that is, anticipating the worst and being vigilant for signs of danger. They may engage in repetitive thinking or brooding, known as rumination. In addition, they may experience a whole range of distressing physical symptoms (e.g., gastrointestinal symptoms like nausea and diarrhea, sweating, heart palpitations, dizziness, hot flushes, or cold chills) and emotional states (e.g., apprehension or dread, tension, restlessness, irritability). See Exhibit 4.1 for a list of anxiety disorders most common in young adults.

It is important to note that the symptoms of several types of anxiety disorders can mimic medical conditions such as asthma, hyperthyroidism, and adrenal dysfunction, making a correct diagnosis difficult. Further complicating the diagnostic process are those situations when alcohol and/or drug use is excessive and actually contributes to the development of anxiety disorders. We say more about this in Chapter 6.

For an emerging adult who is experiencing more serious anxiety, the prospect of taking an upcoming exam or participating in a job interview may produce feelings of dread, negative thoughts, and physical symptoms. Irritability and annoyance even over little

---

EXHIBIT 4.1. Anxiety Disorders Common in Young Adults

Generalized Anxiety Disorder
- Excessive worry
- Worry that feels out of control

Panic Disorder
- Presence of panic attacks (i.e., pounding heart, shortness of breath, shaking, sweating, fear of going crazy, etc.)
- Constant worry about having another panic attack

Social Anxiety
- Fear of negative judgment by others
- Fears lead to limited social contact or isolation

things are also commonly seen in young adults with severe anxiety. You will likely observe a decrease in appetite and some weight loss in emerging adults with more serious anxiety. Your emerging adult may have extreme difficulty falling or staying asleep and may consequently experience tiredness and fatigue.

It is common for people with anxiety disorders to engage in distinct patterns of dysfunctional behaviors to cope with the uncomfortable physical sensations, feelings, and thoughts associated with anxiety. Your adult child may engage in avoidant behaviors such as deciding to drop a class midsemester rather than comply with the professor's course requirement of oral class presentations. Or your young adult may perpetually overthink social situations and interactions, such as not letting go of a comment made by a friend.

Young adults may overidentify with a diagnosis and attribute everything to this label; in this case, receiving a diagnosis can serve as a relief but can also become an excuse for whatever is not going well. Escaping anxiety through substance misuse, internet misuse (i.e., gaming, gambling), and self-injury are also common ways for emerging adults to deal with anxiety. Alternatively, your young adult may become overly controlling of aspects of their environment or others around them to compensate for feeling out of control with anxiety.

DEPRESSION IN YOUNG ADULTS

Emerging adults experience depression more than any other age group (Goodwin et al., 2022; Villarroel & Terlizzi, 2020) This may come as a surprise to you, but remember the intensity of challenges that await young people as they approach legal emancipation. Unfortunately, parents often misread or downplay depression in their adult children and regard it as "a bad mood" and believe that their young adult just "needs to snap out of it." The reality is that more serious depression is a complex illness consisting of a whole host of symptoms, some of which are physiological, while others are behavioral, cognitive, and emotional in nature. Most people assume that young adults struggling with serious depression are sad, but this is not always the case. Young adults often describe their mood as empty or numb; they may come across as irritable and grouchy or vacant and expressionless. Changes in sleep is another symptom suggesting serious depression. Although it is often difficult to pick up on a change in your adult child's sleep schedule, the change in sleep patterns is quite dramatic when they are dealing with depression. They may either sleep most of the day and night, or, conversely, they might be unable to fall or remain asleep. These sleep disruptions in young adults often result in chronic feelings of fatigue. Additional symptoms may include changes in appetite or weight, loss of concentration, and a decrease in self-esteem, among others. The most concerning symptom of serious depression is thoughts of death or suicide. We discuss suicide in detail later in this chapter. Exhibit 4.2 lists the symptoms of major depressive disorder.

For your young adult to be given a diagnosis of major depressive disorder, these symptoms need to be present for at least 2 weeks

---

EXHIBIT 4.2. Symptoms of Major Depressive Disorder

- Very sad, depressed mood
- Lack of interest in hobbies and activities previously enjoyed
- Change in weight or appetite
- Sleeping, either too much or not enough
- Feeling agitated or slowed down
- Fatigue or loss of energy
- Feeling worthless or guilty
- Difficulty concentrating
- Thoughts of death or suicide

---

and interfere with the ability to perform daily tasks before a diagnosis can be made. Serious depression does not suddenly appear in your adult child; it develops slowly over time as the symptoms begin to infiltrate their thoughts and behaviors. Some symptoms may be easy to miss, especially if you are not having regular contact with your young adult. Once again, it is important to understand that medical disorders such as hypothyroidism, diabetes, and chronic fatigue syndrome, for example, can masquerade as depression, thus complicating the diagnostic process. Similarly, overuse of substances can induce major depressive disorder.

In many young adults, more serious anxiety can coexist along with their depression. For example, in 2023, a national survey found that half of adults aged 18 to 24 reported symptoms of both anxiety and depression compared with only one third of adults (National Center for Health Statistics, 2023). In Chapter 3, Anne's symptoms included both anxiety and depression; it is not uncommon for both these symptoms to be present in young adults. Try to imagine having a mixture of the uncomfortable physical sensations, feelings, and thoughts associated with anxiety while at the same time experiencing the downward spiral of depression. It is no wonder that young adults are drawn to alcohol, drugs, junk food, gaming, and social media dragons as coping tools.

If your emerging adult is struggling with both more serious anxiety and depression, you might notice them withdrawing from friends and family. This could take the form of increased time alone in their room or increased time with technology (e.g., gaming, social media). A word of caution: Using social media is fairly typical in this age group and is not always a sign of serious anxiety and depression. However, if you sense they are avoiding all social activities and interactions, this may be a cause for concern. Your adult child could appear apathetic and spend less time engaging in activities they previously enjoyed and devoted considerable time to, such as sports, music, or reading. Behaviors such as dropping out of school or quitting a job can be red flags for more serious anxiety and depression.

Even when your adult child is no longer living at home, parents can have a "gut feeling" that their young adult is in distress. Frequently, these feelings are accurate. And often parents dismiss these feelings. Even if your adult child may no longer be living in your home, you may still see evidence that they are struggling to concentrate on school or work tasks. They may complain to you about their battle to recall information when preparing for a test or their sudden inability to comprehend what they have read. These difficulties may result in missed or dropped classes, lower grades, more sick days, or poor performance reviews at work. It's important to trust your gut.

WHY DOES MY ADULT CHILD HAVE ANXIETY OR DEPRESSION?

Researchers have found that more serious anxiety and depression are most likely triggered by a combination of biological, psychological, and sociocultural factors converging at just the right time (Korb, 2015; Kwong et al., 2019; Nasir & Lacroix, 2022). Just as scientists now believe there is no single cause of cancer but rather an interaction of many factors (Saini et al., 2020), so are anxiety and depression heterogeneous disorders with multiple underlying causes.

In terms of biological factors, you may have heard that more serious anxiety and depression run in families, meaning some people have a genetic vulnerability to anxiety and depression. If you or your partner/spouse has been diagnosed with a severe anxiety or mood disorder, your young adult's chances of also developing anxiety and depression are higher than they would be in the absence of family history. This tendency toward severe anxiety and depression stems from a group of genes, not a single gene, passed down from one or both parents. Please keep in mind that a diagnosis of severe depression or anxiety, or both, is not inevitable even if such factors are present in your family.

The brain plays a role in both anxiety and depression, but it operates differently in each case. When we are anxious, our brain works in the same way as it does when we are stressed. Think of anxiety as your body's response to the stress you feel when your body perceives a threat—the stress response we discussed in Chapter 1. As we mentioned there, stress is our response to a threat. However, anxiety may not have any trigger at all. In addition, stress tends to be shorter term than anxiety. Symptoms of stress and anxiety are similar—faster heartbeat, faster breathing, feeling overwhelmed, and so on. Regardless of whether your young adult is struggling with stress, anxiety, or both, the role of the brain is much the same.

With depression the role of the brain is less clear. In recent years, researchers have moved away from the theory that a chemical imbalance in the brain causes depression. Rather than viewing depression as having a single cause, it is now believed to be the result of several factors coming into play at the same time: high or chronic levels of stress, changes in hormones, an unhealthy diet, and genetics, among others (Korb, 2015; Owczarek et al., 2022). The research on diet and nutritional deficiencies may eventually prove quite useful because many emerging adults are typically "fast-food" fanatics and not particularly nutrition conscious (Owczarek et al., 2022). When you combine poor diet, sleep deprivation, and a sedentary lifestyle in a young adult, their risk for depression increases significantly.

A number of psychological stressors also contribute to severe anxiety and depression in young adults, including parental dysfunction (incarceration, substance abuse, mental health concerns, etc.) current stressors, loneliness, personal loss experiences, and personality characteristics (Piechaczek et al., 2020; Sayyah et al., 2022). Current stressors can be both positive and negative (e.g., graduation, beginning a new job, the birth of a child, relationship breakup, chronic family conflict, failing out of school, losing a job).

Let's take the example of graduating from high school. For many, turning 18 is a positive experience, at least initially, as they move on to college or work pursuits. At the same time, it can be a scary experience, with changes such as moving away from home to a dorm or apartment, having to meet new people, and taking on new responsibilities without having parents readily available when things get tough. For some young adults, the challenges seem to outweigh the initial euphoria of freedom. Such situations can elicit feelings of anxiety or depression, or both.

Since the COVID-19 pandemic, loneliness has been identified as a psychological factor contributing to anxiety and depression in emerging adults. Social interaction took place through online social platforms rather than in person, and in many cases, the young adult's need for social connection was not met. As recently as 2023, the U.S. Surgeon General (Office of the Surgeon General) identified social isolation as a major factor contributing to mental health issues such as depression.

Without a doubt, loss has the potential to contribute to more serious depression and anxiety. The death of a grandparent or a beloved pet may be your emerging adult's first experience with death. There are many ways your young adult might experience a loss other than through death, such as parents' divorce, relocating due to a parent's job change, or being rejected by those they consider friends. Obviously, some of these losses are more manageable than others. In these situations, your adult child will need to learn about the grieving process and develop coping strategies. In the absence of such strategies, depression and anxiety are likely to get worse.

There are also certain personality traits that can put your adult child more at risk for serious anxiety and depression. Emerging adults who are highly sensitive, self-critical, and lacking in self-esteem may be more prone to severe anxiety and depression than those who are more confident and self-assured. Just as with biological factors, psychological factors do not, in and of themselves, lead to the development of severe anxiety and depression. However, they are red flags that need attention.

Sociocultural factors also contribute to serious anxiety and depression and other serious mental illnesses in emerging adults (Kirkbride et al., 2024), particularly in LGBT persons, persons of color, and other cultural minorities (Williams, 2018). Discrimination, harassment, physical and emotional abuse, victimization, and isolation are experiences associated with race, ethnicity, religion, disability, sexual orientation, and gender nonconformity. Not only are persons in these groups more vulnerable to serious mental illnesses, but they have less access to treatment, and they are frequently misdiagnosed, all of which leads to very poor outcomes. As mentioned earlier, none of these factors alone will trigger symptoms of severe depression or anxiety, but when combined with psychological factors and one's level of biological vulnerability, the likelihood of developing a mood disorder increases.

BIPOLAR DISORDERS IN YOUNG ADULTS

Clinicians use the term *bipolar spectrum* to describe numerous types of bipolar disorders including bipolar I, bipolar II, and cyclothymia, among others. For our purposes here, we focus on the two most serious disorders: bipolar I and bipolar II disorder.

Bipolar I Disorder

You have undoubtedly heard of bipolar disorder or manic depression when describing someone whose mood fluctuates like a roller coaster. Think about bipolar disorder as one of extremes with depression at one end or pole and mania at the opposite end or pole. Exhibit 4.3 lists symptoms of mania in bipolar I disorder.

EXHIBIT 4.3. Symptoms of Mania in Bipolar I Disorder

- Extremely high self-esteem
- Going full-speed with little or no sleep
- Talking way more than usual
- Thoughts racing a mile a minute
- Very easily distracted
- Highly ambitious and goal-directed activity; super productive
- Restless, agitated, fidgety
- Participating in high-risk activities with potential harmful outcome

---

People with bipolar I disorder have at least one manic episode that lasts a minimum of 1 week. A depressive episode may or may not have been present before the manic episode. An episode of mania is essential before a diagnosis of bipolar I can be made. Symptoms of mania are hard to miss, particularly if you are witnessing your young adult's manic episode for the first time. If your emerging adult is in the midst of a manic episode, you will notice a radical change in their behavior. Your adult child might act like they are on top of the world, and nothing can stop them! Mania is experienced in emerging adults as a high, a time of frenetic activity and boundless energy. They can't seem to stop talking, texting, and phoning; they can't focus on anything for more than a few minutes. Young adults feel overly exuberant, like "superman," and act like they are "multitasking on steroids." They may go without sleep for several days. Although manic episodes can yield remarkable accomplishments in the short run, such as writing a term paper overnight or painting your studio apartment in an afternoon, the end result is most always the same: The emerging adult crashes.

During a manic episode, young adults can be agitated and unreasonable, openly combative, and aggressive, without tolerance for anyone. Left untreated bipolar I disorder can lead to aggressive and destructive behaviors aimed at self and others, particularly during mania, mixed episodes, and when psychotic symptoms are present. Mixed episodes refer to a period of time when symptoms of depression and mania, or hypomania, are present. (Hypomania is described in the next section on bipolar II disorder.) Your emerging adult may go on a shopping spree, spending money on things they don't need and cannot afford, a common occurrence during this mood state. They may also engage in high-risk behaviors like driving recklessly, becoming hypersexual and engaging in unsafe sexual behaviors, excessively using drugs and alcohol, gaming, and gambling. They may self-injure by cutting themselves or burning their body with cigarettes. And they are generally impervious to perceptions of others who view them as out of control.

Manic episodes are sometimes accompanied by psychotic symptoms including delusions, such as unrealistic, bizarre, and paranoid beliefs that others are spying on or plotting against them. We use the term *psychotic symptoms* to refer to a loss of touch with reality (e.g., feeling like others are out to get you with no evidence that it is true). The other classic symptom of psychosis is hallucinations that involve sensory experiences, such as seeing things that don't exist or hearing voices that aren't real. For example, your adult child may confide in you that she "hears birds speaking gibberish" and may hear an outside voice that says, "No one likes you and you should die." These symptoms are frightening for the young adult, and also the parent, when they occur.

As stated earlier, psychotic symptoms can appear in major depressive disorder as well as bipolar disorder. It is vital, however, that providers consider alternative explanations for psychosis first, including use of certain medications and substance misuse (e.g., alcohol, cocaine, methamphetamine, ecstasy) before attributing the symptoms to bipolar disorder or major depressive disorder.

Bipolar II Disorder

Bipolar II is often described as a less intense form of bipolar I, but to a large extent, this is untrue because bipolar II disorder can present in a very different way. Bipolar II also involves mood fluctuations between depression and hypomania. The term *hypomania* is used to describe a lesser form of mania and is discussed in detail shortly. An individual with bipolar II disorder typically experiences more depression, and the duration of the depressive episodes can be quite long with considerable impairment in daily functioning. The depressive episodes of bipolar II disorder are often characterized by the less typical aspects of depression, such as psychomotor agitation (i.e., restlessness or pacing), feelings of guilt, increased weight and appetite, fear of rejection, and increased need for sleep.

The symptoms of hypomania are virtually the same as the symptoms of mania, but they are of shorter duration and involve less risk. In addition, the symptoms only need to be present for 4 consecutive days to qualify as an episode of hypomania. Young adults may experience certain hypomanic symptoms as pleasant and desirable, especially at first. For example, feeling a heightened sense of self-confidence and the belief that all things are possible, they may take on too many projects. In a hypomanic episode, potential risks are minimized or ignored, and the immediate priority is fun. It is not uncommon for young adults with a diagnosis of bipolar II to experience frustration, perceive others as "stupid" or "annoying," and to engage in arguments or disagreements when experiencing hypomania.

The Challenge of Diagnosing Bipolar Disorder

It should be clear from what you have read so far that bipolar disorder is a highly complex illness, and as a result, making an accurate diagnosis is quite challenging. Researchers have found the delay from the first appearance of symptoms to the time of diagnosis can range from 5 to 11 years (Baldessarini et al., 2003; Keramatian et al., 2022; Medici et al., 2015). Because bipolar illness often looks like depression early on, emerging adults are frequently misdiagnosed with major depressive disorder and ultimately treated with the wrong medication—medication that could actually intensify or worsen the symptoms associated with bipolar disorder. Early signs of mania or hypomania are often missed as the medical provider is often more focused on depression.

Unfortunately, it takes time for "bipolar depression" to swing from depression toward symptoms of mania or hypomania. Some factors that could signal a possible swing toward mania include having an early-onset episode of depression (beginning early in life) with the episode being of short duration and coming to a sudden end, a recurrent pattern, poor response to antidepressants, and a family history of bipolar disorder. To complicate matters further, other mental health conditions are sometimes confused with bipolar disorder (e.g., attention-deficit/hyperactivity disorder, borderline personality disorder, schizophrenia, anxiety disorders). In some cases, these disorders are even diagnosed alongside bipolar disorder.

Interestingly there are also medical conditions such as thyroid disease and multiple sclerosis that can masquerade as bipolar disorder and complicate the diagnostic process. Additionally, certain medications (e.g., decongestants, prescription pain medications, antidepressants) have been found to induce symptoms of bipolar disorder. It's easy to understand why bipolar disorder often takes years to diagnose. Should you be considering help for your young adult, we recommend finding a psychiatric provider highly trained to diagnose serious mental illnesses, such as bipolar disorder, in emerging adults. The provider will evaluate your adult child's specific symptoms, timeframes, severity, and the degree to which day-to-day functioning is impaired before making a diagnosis. Information regarding the training and credentials of mental health providers will be provided in Chapter 6.

Let's hear once again from Claire, Anne's mother:

> After Anne turned 19, I noticed she withdrew more and didn't communicate much with her dad and me. When she finally did come to me and share that she felt anxious and depressed, I listened with empathy and concern. I probably should have stopped there instead of offering my advice and urging her to see a therapist. One day to my surprise, Anne told me she made an appointment with her family nurse practitioner. I was relieved to know that Anne was getting help. However, Anne shared very few details of her treatment with me, except when she complained about her medication. In retrospect I think she felt so badly, so unlike herself, that she couldn't help but say something. It worried me that most of the time, Anne wouldn't talk to me at all. There were many times when she angrily reminded me she was over 18 and didn't need to share any information about herself with me anymore.
>
> Within the first 6 months of starting treatment with her nurse practitioner, I noticed that Anne was behaving in ways that were very atypical of her. It was horrific when we received a call from the police that Anne was found wandering the downtown area. She was disheveled, disoriented, and agitated. She claimed to believe that she was Katniss Everdeen, the lead character from the Hunger Games series. The police accompanied her to the ER, at which point the on-call psychiatrist diagnosed her as having bipolar disorder, admitted her to the inpatient psychiatric unit, and ultimately changed her medication.

Often, parents may have a very different reaction to their young adult's situation, and this is true for Claire and Stan. Listen to Stan's perception of what is happening with his daughter:

> Anne always talked more with her mother than with me. I thought that Claire was blowing things out of proportion. I was never as

concerned about Anne as she was. I just assumed what Anne was going through was typical coming-of-age stuff, no big deal. Boy, was I wrong! But now that we have a diagnosis, I feel better. There is medicine that will help Anne. We have a plan to move forward. I keep trying to tell Claire that, but she's always been too protective of Anne. She has a really hard time letting go. Sure, I'm worried too, but we have to keep this thing in perspective.

Claire and Stan's story is frightening for any parent to hear and shows how parents may react to a situation in very different ways. It also underscores the challenges associated with getting an accurate diagnosis and the correct medication. An inexperienced practitioner may miss the early signs associated with bipolar illness and, as a result, treat young adults with the wrong medication—medication that could actually intensify the symptoms associated with bipolar disorder. In Anne's case, her manic state was the result of misdiagnosis and perhaps treatment with the wrong medication, which in turn led to her emergency hospitalization. We devote the next two chapters to addressing steps that you, as a parent, might take to lessen the chances of this happening to your young adult. In Chapter 6, we present key information and strategies about how to deal with a young adult who is resistant to your involvement in their treatment.

WHY DOES MY ADULT CHILD HAVE BIPOLAR DISORDER?

Bipolar disorder is a multifaceted disorder with a strong hereditary component. In plain English, this means both biological and psychological factors contribute to the development of the disorder. As is true for severe depression, there is no one cause of bipolar disorder, although scientists agree that family history is the best predictor of this mental illness. Young adults whose parent or sibling has been diagnosed with bipolar disorder are more at risk for the disorder than are those with no family history. This is especially true if symptoms first appeared in the parent or sibling just before or soon after puberty. Additional biologically based risk factors include a chemical imbalance of the neurotransmitters or chemical messengers in the brain as well as possible abnormalities in the physical structure of the brain. Even if there is a history of bipolar disorder in your family, keep in mind it is not inevitable that your young adult will develop bipolar disorder.

Psychological factors with the potential to increase your adult child's vulnerability to bipolar disorder include high stress, a history of trauma, significant losses, sleep deprivation, and substance abuse. Unfortunately, substance use and sleep loss are common in emerging adults, making it difficult to determine whether concern is warranted. Sleep deprivation is common among young adults whether it be due to inconsistent work hours or spending all night on social media. Regardless of the reason, changes in the sleep–wake cycle should be monitored as sleep deprivation is a key symptom of bipolar disorder.

Relative to substance use, emerging adults with undiagnosed bipolar disorder may choose to use or abuse substances in their efforts to manage their distressing and disruptive symptoms. Using substances to cope with undiagnosed bipolar symptoms is common among young adults. Substance abuse does not cause bipolar disorder, but it could quicken the onset of symptoms, worsen mood episodes, and complicate the diagnostic process. Additionally, if your adult child uses substances long enough before a diagnosis of bipolar disorder is given, they could also receive a diagnosis of substance abuse disorder.

As with severe anxiety and depression, experiences of discrimination, harassment, abuse, and so forth are common among persons of color or other minority groups. Such experiences may serve to increase one's vulnerability to bipolar disorder. However, it is essential to remember there is no absolute formula to predict who will and who will not develop bipolar disorder.

WHAT TO DO IF YOUR ADULT CHILD HAS DEPRESSION, ANXIETY, OR BIPOLAR DISORDER

For many parents, the onset of mental health disorders in their adult children is the equivalent of what Bruce Feiler (2020) termed a "lifequake." It most certainly can be an experience that destroys your sense of stability and may leave you feeling disoriented and completely vulnerable. The aftermath of this new reality creates aftershocks that may be felt for years. It is important for you to be able to stay on relatively even footing as you work through this lifequake, employing the tools of a coach, such as emotional regulation and empathy (for yourself and your adult child). It is also important to monitor your own stress and use breathing techniques in the moment when you feel the tension rising. At the risk of sounding like a broken record, the breathing exercises we offer throughout the book are your frontline defense in high stress situations. They are free, and you can use them almost anywhere.

Watching your adult child struggle with symptoms of more serious mental illnesses is obviously extremely difficult and can prompt a variety of reactions. As a parent, you may find yourself minimizing your adult child's depression and anxiety. You may be tempted to try to talk your emerging adult out of worry, rumination, and depression. Unfortunately, this often only serves to intensify these symptoms. Educating yourself about mental disorders can be a way of reducing your stress and feeling more empowered in your interactions with your adult child.

For some parents, their emerging adults' symptoms overshadow the rest of the family members' needs, resulting in parents' remorse about not giving their other children time and much-needed attention. Other parents may be completely unaware of these dynamics and what may be happening with the rest of the family. We talk more in Chapter 7 about the family system.

Another predominant reaction for many parents is guilt and self-blame. These feelings can be intense as parents begin to grapple with the possibility that their young adult has serious anxiety or depression. Parents wonder "what if" and "how" they have "failed" their adult child. These self-attacking thoughts and accompanying feelings of regret can be even more magnified when parents themselves have struggled with depression, anxiety, or other mental health issues such as substance misuse.

It is important for parents to recognize the parallel process they and their adult children experience. Both emerging adults and their parents are faced with a lot of uncertainty about the future and are often concerned about the impact a mental health diagnosis could have on the young adult's record (e.g., difficulty being admitted to a university, being turned down by the military). These concerns may contribute to the adult child's reluctance or outright refusal to seek treatment. Unfortunately, when parents are unable either to convince their young adults to seek therapy or to assist them in navigating the mental health system, many report feelings of frustration and helplessness. It is the case for many parents that the only way their adult child can get psychiatric treatment is if they are in a crisis. This means that they are a risk to themselves or others. Parents are stuck in a waiting game while they witness their adult child's deterioration. Tragically, the longer the delays in obtaining treatment, the greater the potential for both symptoms and overall prognosis to worsen. In Chapter 6, we offer useful strategies for parents dealing with resistance to mental health treatment often verbalized by young adults. For now, though, remember to breathe and use the information you have learned to keep your emotions from overwhelming you.

Although the appearance of symptoms of any mental illness in your adult child may freak you out, behaviors reflective of bipolar disorder, specifically bipolar I, may feel most alarming because this illness can significantly hinder your young adult's progress toward important milestones. As we stated earlier, bipolar illness is one of the more complicated mental health disorders, and unfortunately it often begins during the emerging-adult phase of life. It is essential to note that no two cases of bipolar disorder ever appear the same, which adds to the challenge of making an accurate diagnosis. However, a proactive response to the symptoms improves the potential for them to be managed.

That being said, should your adult child receive a diagnosis of bipolar I disorder, it is typical to respond with shock and denial, followed by sadness and despair. Early on, many parents try to attribute changes or symptoms in their young adult to other factors such as substance misuse, rarely getting enough sleep, or living an unhealthy lifestyle. However, these explanations typically don't hold up for very long. This is especially true if you witnessed your young adult during a manic episode in which they were unable to differentiate between reality and the hallucinations or delusions they were experiencing.

Parents typically fear that a serious mental illness means the end of their adult child's educational and employment goals, social networks, and ability to sustain a long-term relationship and establish a family. The loss of a predictable trajectory for the life of your adult child is quite troubling for most parents. It might be the first time parents ever experienced a loss of this nature, a loss of all the things parents assumed would transpire in the lives of their young adults. We will talk a lot more about loss and grief as it relates to serious mental illness in Chapter 8.

At age 16, Elyn Saks (2008) who authored the book *The Center Cannot Hold: My Journey Through Madness*, was diagnosed with severe mental illness and given a poor prognosis by her doctors. Now the author, mental health advocate, and law professor at the University of Southern California, says, "I needed to put two critical ideas together: that I could both be mentally ill and lead a rich and satisfying life" (Saks, 2008, p. 133). It is your job as coach to take this idea to heart: It can be possible to have a full life even with a mental health disorder. Allow this possibility to guide you as you continue your journey with your adult child.

In addition to trying to manage the range of psychological issues with your young adult, whether they stem from anxiety, depression, or bipolar disorder, your communication with them has likely been highly charged and even volatile. Not only does this add to your stress, but there is a potential for your young adult to become physically aggressive and threaten your safety. The parent who experiences symptoms of trauma at the same time their emerging adult is exhibiting symptoms of a serious mental illness, is under duress and needs support. In Chapter 9, we discuss the necessity of pivoting in these instances to your own self-care.

As for helping your adult child when they have depression, anxiety, or bipolar disorder, this likely involves learning some additional skills that are associated with the advanced coach role. We discuss these skills in detail in the next chapter.

This might be a good time to add another breathing exercise to your tote bag as we prepare to deal with the topic of suicide. Please consult Exhibit 4.4.

 SUICIDAL THOUGHTS, BEHAVIORS, AND ATTEMPTS IN YOUNG ADULTS

Let's return to the story of Daniel first introduced in the introduction chapter and hear from his father Arturo:

> Daniel seemed to be doing well with his grades and his friends
> at college until the first semester of his sophomore year when

EXHIBIT 4.4. **Calming Exercise: Alternate Nostril Breathing**

Place your thumb on your right nostril. With this nostril covered, close your eyes and exhale fully and slowly through your left nostril. Once you've exhaled completely, release your right nostril and put your ring finger on the left nostril. Breathe in deeply and slowly from the right side. Repeat this exercise five to ten times.

his girlfriend, Alessandra, broke up with him. I remember sometime after that I kept asking him over and over for his team schedule. I wanted to try to get to a couple of his games. He kept making excuses . . . like he didn't have it with him. He kept promising to get it to me. Finally, I'm at work one day and I get a call from his coach, who had recruited Daniel and even came to watch him in high school. Real good guy. . . . He starts telling me Daniel's missing practices and he's hearing back from some of his professors that he's missing classes too. I come home that night and tell my wife and the next thing you know she's calling Daniel asking what's going on? He starts crying and says he isn't doing well. He pleads to come home. We were so shocked. He just kept saying, "I can't take any more. I just want to close my eyes and disappear."

The next day, my wife is on the phone calling the university. She talks to someone who tells her he needs to go to the university counseling center and the academic advising office. She manages to talk Daniel into seeing a counselor, who says he has got bad depression and anxiety. He still says he wants to come home. So, my wife calls the university and figures out how to get a leave of absence for Daniel. We drove up to the university to move him home the next day.

What did you think as you read about Daniel? How did you feel about how Daniel's parents responded to their son's depression?

Did Daniel's statement, "I can't take any more. I just want to close my eyes and disappear," raise red flags for you?

Much to our collective alarm, the rates of suicidal attempts and suicidal deaths among adolescents and young adults is increasing. According to the latest findings from the Centers for Disease Control and Prevention (2020), suicide in the United States was the second leading cause of death for young adults. The recent annual percentage of young adults in the United States trying to end their lives is 1 in 50.

Young adults who are diagnosed with either severe depression or bipolar disorder are especially at risk for suicidal thoughts and behaviors. Suicidal thoughts can occur during mood episodes such as depression, mania, hypomania, and during psychotic states. One-third of suicide attempts by persons with bipolar disorder take place in the first year after the onset of symptoms (Salvatore et al., 2007). This is cause for concern and highlights the importance of early and effective treatment.

Suicidal thoughts can come and go, or they can be constantly running through the person's mind. They can also feel intrusive or be welcomed by that person. *Passive* suicidal thoughts include wishing to die or not waking up in the morning, while *active* thoughts include, for example, wanting to kill oneself and having a detailed plan in mind. Recently, researchers have begun to explore the possibility that some people experience visual images of suicide in addition to just thinking about it (Lawrence et al., 2022). In other words, they literally visualize images of themselves making a suicide attempt. These images, termed *suicidal flash-forwards*, allow the individual to rehearse their own suicide and thereby become more comfortable with the idea of dying. In addition, there is evidence to suggest that these suicidal flashforwards indicate a greater likelihood of making suicidal plans and actually attempting suicide rather than just thinking or talking about suicide (De Rozario et al., 2021).

WHY DOES MY ADULT CHILD EXHIBIT SUICIDAL THOUGHTS, BEHAVIORS, OR ATTEMPTS?

Researchers known as suicidologists study data about suicide and self-harm to help prevent suicide. They identify numerous risk factors that increase the likelihood that a person will experience suicidal thoughts and behaviors as well as protective factors that reduce the likelihood of attempting or completing suicide. When assessing for suicide risk, mental health professionals consider these risk and protective factors and ask whether an individual has active suicidal thoughts, detailed plans, and access to lethal means.

The presence of mental illness (e.g., severe depression, bipolarity, anxiety, substance use) and physical health issues (e.g., chronic illness and pain, disabilities, traumatic brain injury) increase the potential for suicide attempts and completions. Social factors such as a lack of supportive relationships with others (e.g., being rejected; being in a violent or high-conflict relationship; being harassed, bullied, or cyberbullied) and various losses (e.g., the end of a relationship) are considered factors that increase the potential risk for suicide. In addition, socioeconomic disadvantages such as discrimination, marginalization, and homelessness contribute to increased risk for suicide. For example, rates of suicidal thinking and suicide attempts among young LGBT adults are higher than among their heterosexual peers (Salway et al., 2021). Multiple stressors such as victimization, rejection, and stigma significantly contribute to suicidal ideation or thinking and attempts among LGBT young adults.

Psychological risk factors that are associated with suicidal ideation are impulsiveness, perfectionism, hopelessness, perceived burdensomeness to others, self-hatred, and shame. These feelings can reach intolerable levels, and young adults may become focused on suicide as the only means of ridding themselves of their emotional pain. Thinking about suicide can be a means of coping as well as a form of distraction from painful emotions. Some young adults spend hours visualizing and planning their suicide and the aftermath of their death. Prior exposure to suicide (e.g., that of a relative or friend) or a previous history of suicidal thoughts and behaviors together with self-injury, can numb a young adult to pain and death. It is important to keep in mind that many young adults haven't lived long enough to understand that the sun comes up tomorrow. For many, life is here and now, so when a relationship ends, there's no thought that another one is or may be waiting in the future somewhere. This is the one and only, and if it ends, all hope is lost. Such thinking leaves many young adults vulnerable to the risk of suicide.

Alternately, protective factors include positive coping and decision-making strategies, spiritual beliefs that discourage suicide, positive life satisfaction, and having goals and dreams. External protective factors include multiple forms of social support such as family ties, friendships, a positive therapeutic relationship, and other resources for healing such as yoga and meditation. Additionally, engaging in activities that help others, including pets, can be a protective factor for young adults.

 ## WHAT TO DO IF YOUR ADULT CHILD EXHIBITS SUICIDAL THOUGHTS, BEHAVIORS, OR ATTEMPTS

Many adult children are hesitant to share suicidal thoughts with their parents and other family members because of fears of being ridiculed, criticized, belittled, or hospitalized. In some cases, parents may have established family rules that downplay or discourage the expression of negative emotions. It is also possible that your young adult may not disclose their suicidal thoughts to anyone. However, they may make comments such as "I hate my life," "I want to disappear," or "If only I could go to sleep and never wake up."

Parents get anxious about asking their adult child about suicidal thoughts. Some parents fear that by raising the issue of suicide, they will plant the idea and upset their young adult. One way to begin this important but difficult dialogue with your adult child is by saying "a lot of people who go through this experience and feel so miserable sometimes wish they were dead. Do you ever think about killing yourself?" By putting the topic out there, you in effect invite your adult child to talk about what they are feeling and/or thinking without judgment. It is scary to think about and even harder to actually say the words to them. Very often it is also what opens the door to talking about what they are going through and assisting them in getting the help they need.

The aftermath of a young adult's suicide attempt is nothing short of a nightmare for parents. The shock and terror for parents is often jarring. Your young adult's decision to seek hospitalization related to a suicide attempt is an extraordinarily difficult one. If they are involuntarily hospitalized because they are considered, by a qualified mental health professional, to be in imminent danger of dying by suicide, this experience will likely be distressing and unpleasant both for them and for you. Hospital stays average less than 1 week, and in many cases, the primary mode of therapy is group counseling. An important aspect of your adult child's inpatient treatment entails establishing a safety plan.

A parent can quickly become laser-focused on keeping their young adult alive. Life as you know it comes to a grinding halt as the mission of keeping your young adult safe becomes your goal. In addition, many parents as well as other family members, exhibit signs of secondary trauma (e.g., nightmares and sleep disruption, intrusive thoughts, being constantly on guard) in response to their young adult's suicide attempt. Some parents may also experience their young adult's suicidal behavior as a "rupture" of relationship and feel a sense of anger and betrayal. While you are focused on helping your adult child, it is essential that you monitor your own well-being and work to reduce your anxiety.

In addition, parents further worry about the risks of future suicidal behavior. Your adult child is especially vulnerable during the period immediately after an unsuccessful suicide attempt. Approximately 15% of those who attempt suicide will try again within 6 months (B. P. Liu et al., 2020). Particularly in the early stages after their adult child's suicide attempt, parents often engage in the process of ruminating on the question of "why?" In her book, *Never Let Go: How to Parent Your Child Through Mental Illness*, Alderson (2020) described the inevitable stream of self-incriminating thoughts and questions she and other parents experienced in the wake of their child's suicidal thoughts and behaviors (e.g., "Why didn't we see this coming?," "What didn't we do?," "I was too busy working," "I should never have gotten remarried"). These questions are an automatic or reflexive response and so is the ruminating. In Chapter 8, we discuss in more detail ways in which parents can deal with the significant grief and other reactions that occur when your emerging adult engages in self-harm and suicidal behavior.

Relationships with partners are often affected when a young adult struggles with suicidal thinking and behavior. Marriages become strained and communication is disrupted. Siblings are also affected. Their reactions include anger, resentment, and frustration, as well as the desire to help and support their brother or sister. In Chapter 5 we discuss ways in which family members can be negatively impacted (called *collateral damage*) and offer recommendations for how parents can intervene.

SELF-INJURY IN YOUNG ADULTS

One form of managing emotional distress, particularly in young adults, is nonsuicidal self-injury. Young adults are considered a population at-risk for nonsuicidal self-injury, and these behaviors are often mingled with symptoms of other mental health disorders including anxiety, major depressive disorder, bipolar disorder, substance use, and eating disorders. Such behaviors are defined as deliberate, intentional actions that result in damage to the body and occur without the intent to end one's own life. These behaviors can entail cutting, severely scratching or biting oneself, carving into the skin, burning oneself with a cigarette, inserting objects under the skin or nails, and punching oneself to the point of bruising and bleeding. Typically, these behaviors begin in adolescence and vary in frequency and intensity. The increased demands associated with the emerging adult stage provoke a spike in self-injurious behaviors.

Nonsuicidal self-injury was first included as a disorder in the *Diagnostic and Statistical Manual of Mental Disorders*, fourth edition, text revision (*DSM-IV-TR*; American Psychiatric Association, 2000) as an area for future study. According to the diagnostic criteria, these behaviors must occur for a minimum of 5 days in a period of 1 year. Tattoos and body piercing are not considered examples of self-injurious behaviors because they are socially and culturally acceptable practices. However, some mental health experts (e.g., Whitlock & Lloyd-Richardson, 2019) view nonsuicidal self-injury as a growing concern among youth and cite the impact of the rising popularity of body modification practices as well as social media as possible contributing factors to the increase in self-injury.

There are multiple risks of nonsuicidal self-injury, including scarring, infection, severe bleeding, tissue damage, anemia, and accidental death. Ironically, the distress that is created by engaging in these behaviors only increases feelings of shame, guilt, and distress in your young adult and can contribute to the development of other mental health disorders, such as anxiety disorders.

Young adults engage in nonsuicidal self-injurious behaviors for a variety of reasons, such as the need to distract from or manage intense negative emotions (e.g., sadness, anger, anxiety), a desire to regain a sense of reality in response to periods where one feels disconnected from reality, and as a means of addressing numbness. For some young adults, nonsuicidal self-injury may be a cry for help. Nonsuicidal self-injury actually functions as a coping mechanism, although not a healthy one. Negative emotion can feel overwhelming and out of control, particularly for those who struggle to name and regulate their emotions. The act of intentionally harming the body in some way often creates a sense of control. Additionally intense negative emotion is often difficult to put into words, which serves only to heighten or strengthen the emotion.

An injury to the body offers the young adult something specific to focus on, i.e., a physical injury with the appearance of blood and the feeling of pain. It is often easier for the adult child to focus on the pain and appearance of a physical injury than it is for them to name and manage negative emotion. The goal is not to harm the body but to ground and calm the mind. Those most prone to nonsuicidal self-injury have often been victims of childhood and adolescent trauma such as sexual, physical, and emotional abuse; neglect, family conflict and loss; and having a parent with mental health challenges.

It is important to note that a prior history of self-injurious behavior can be a risk factor for suicide. Repeated self-cutting can result in a serious unintentional injury or accidental death. However, these behaviors are more typically associated with the desire to feel better and not to end one's life. Young adults are able to access information about how to self-harm on the internet. Members of the LGBTQ community and persons such as immigrants and refugees are particularly at risk for self-injury due to the increased level of stress they experience daily just for being themselves (R. T. Liu et al., 2019).

Evidence of self-injury can be hard to detect for a number of reasons. The fresh wounds and scars are often in covered areas of the body and in many cases, your young adult lives away from home or you are not in regular contact. Using clothing, such as long sleeve shirts, to conceal the evidence makes it difficult for others to know what's really going on.

WHAT TO DO IF YOUR ADULT CHILD SELF-INJURES

For parents, the discovery that their young adult child is inflicting physical self-harm can be devastating. Parents are often stunned and terrified. The stress and anxiety related to their young adult's self-harm behavior can contribute to the parent's own anxiety, depression, and physical health problems, including sleeplessness and weight loss. Remember to breathe, coach!

The heightened stress and constant vigilance for signs of potential self-harm create negative reverberations throughout the family. Even when a young person has not self-harmed for some time, parents experience uncertainty about whether it might recur in response to new crises. Parents often experience a sense of "walking on eggshells," as they worry about doing or saying something that might precipitate an episode of self-harm. Siblings also experience similar worries about inadvertently saying or doing something that might trigger self-injury.

Warning signs associated with nonsuicidal self-injury can include suspicious looking wounds and scars, drops of blood, evidence of paraphernalia including hidden razors, knives, other sharp objects, and rubber bands (need to stem blood flow). Quite often young adults who engage in self-injurious behaviors spend long periods of time alone, particularly in the bathroom or bedroom, and wear clothing inappropriate for the weather, such as long sleeves or pants in hot weather.

Talking with your adult child about self-injury is very difficult for most parents. Sometimes parents err on the side of wanting to respond with control rather than support. When you talk with your adult child, it is likely to trigger intense emotional reactions for both you and your young adult. The need to remain calm and nonjudgmental even during emotionally charged situations is essential. And this is not an easy thing to do. Dig into your tote bag and pull out the coach skills you learned in Chapter 2 such as careful listening, emotional regulation, and empathy to help you communicate more effectively in this situation. For example, you are sitting with your adult child when you notice scarring on their lower arm. You notice an intense rise in your anxiety level, and the urge rises to blurt out your thoughts. However, you remind yourself of the importance of taking time to calm yourself and to plan what you would like to say. It is crucial that your tone of voice be calm and supportive and that you speak slowly and softly. You might begin by asking your young adult to share with you how they got the scars. Depending on what they say, you might describe your impressions of the scars, for example, they look concerning to you. You may share your awareness of self-cutting and your understanding that it could stem from some emotional pain and distress. Invite your adult child to talk with you about what they are experiencing.

The capacity to understand and cope with the significant stress associated with nonsuicidal self-injury and to communicate effectively with your young adult will require equipping yourself with a new skill set as an advanced coach. In the next chapter, we describe in detail what the role of the advance coach will entail.

A PARENT'S DILEMMA

When your adult child exhibits the signs and symptoms of a more serious mental health disorder, as a parent, you instinctively want to resume a caretaking role. Regardless of whether your child wants this, you are likely to feel a strong pull to take charge. It is not easy under these circumstances to consider a shift in a new direction. In this chapter, we have provided a wealth of information as a starting point for you to educate yourself about your young adult's mental health issue. This is the first skill in the repertoire of advanced coaching skills that may be especially useful to you when you suspect that your adult child has signs of more serious mental health issues. In the next chapter, we introduce additional advanced coaching skills that will be helpful if your emerging adult has a more serious mental health concern.

Claire, Stan, Arturo, and Lucia are all struggling with the many changes in their emerging adults' mental health. They are observing moods and behaviors they never witnessed before, and they are scared. They will benefit from educating themselves with knowledge about their respective adult child's diagnosed illness. Knowledge is crucial; it increases self-confidence and the ability to ask questions confidently and make sound decisions. Empowerment through knowledge is not one step and done; rather, it is a lifelong learning process. Albert Einstein once described himself as "passionately curious"; he developed an almost childlike wonder for new ideas and information (Pinkowski, 2017, para. 1). Perhaps we, too, can open ourselves to new ideas and information. The more each parent can understand about their adult child's mental health disorder and its impact, the more comfortable and capable they will feel as they navigate these uncharted waters.

SUMMARY

In this chapter, we added to the coaching tools in your tote bag with the skill of educating yourself. We provided a picture of the ways in which severe anxiety, depression, and other related mental illnesses impact the lives of young adults and their parents. We examined the stigma associated with these mental health disorders and discussed the ramifications for parents. Additionally, we identified factors that lessen or intensify the experience for parents. Bipolar disorders are especially difficult to diagnose and are often mistaken for other disorders. This is unfortunate because the key to a more promising prognosis is early treatment. Treatment decreases future mood episodes and reduces the degree of disability or impairment that results from these disorders.

In the next chapter, we provide suggestions to strengthen your existing skills and we offer new skills for your role as advanced coach. We also help you equip yourself emotionally and behaviorally to deal effectively with the demands you face. These demands are challenging! However, the advanced coaching skills will help you strengthen your relationship with your young adult and fortify you for the journey ahead.

POINTS TO POCKET

- Good to know and tough to hear: Individuals are more vulnerable to developing mental disorders during emerging adulthood than at any other time in their lives.
- Listen up: There are many factors that contribute to the development of a mental health disorder. Even if there is a genetic link, you are not responsible.
- "Hope floats." If your adult child has an anxiety and/or mood disorder, there is hope with accurate and timely diagnosis and effective treatment.
- Remember: Listen and support your young adult. Even if you can't understand it, refrain from judging or minimizing their experience.
- Ask the question: If you are concerned about your young adult's safety, ask about self-harm and suicide. It's hard to have this conversation, but it may save their life.

CHAPTER 5

ADVANCED SKILLS FOR SERIOUS MENTAL HEALTH ISSUES

*Always remember, you are braver than you believe, stronger
than you seem, and smarter than you think.*
—Carter & Geurs, *Pooh's Grand Adventure*

This is a good time to stop and take another deep breath. In addition
to becoming equipped with new information, you likely received a
jolt or two from what you read in the previous chapter. The idea that
your young adult might be struggling with a serious mental illness
can overwhelm and frighten you. Perhaps your young adult is dealing with a serious mental health disorder as well as using one of the
dragons to try to cope, and the dragons have become excessive and
dangerous. Or perhaps your young adult has an additional mental
health issue that overlaps with their anxiety or depression, such as
a learning disorder or attention-deficit/hyperactivity disorder
(ADHD). Either way, the combination of more than one concern
can create chaos for both of you. Your adult child's developmental
path is often dramatically altered or even derailed. Education or
career plans may be shelved, and social and romantic relationships
disrupted. The trajectory of their lives no longer seems predictable. As
a parent, your hopes and dreams for your young adult's future, as well
as your own, seem to evaporate. Two sets of our parents—Claire and
Stan and Lucia and Arturo—embody this sense of instability and loss
of direction for the future. Like them, you may experience a range of
emotions from devastation and despair to guilt and anger when your
young adult struggles with mental health issues.

Many parents, yourself included perhaps, will have to transition to advanced coach due to your adult child's more severe form of psychological distress and limited ability to function. In such circumstances, the enhanced skills we present in this chapter will serve as useful tools while you navigate through the difficult challenges ahead. In the Introduction, we presented the parent pivoting wheel in Figure 1. We now offer a modified pivoting wheel in Figure 5.1 which illustrates the advanced coach as an expansion of the coach role (not a new pivot). This expanded role is intended to provide tools

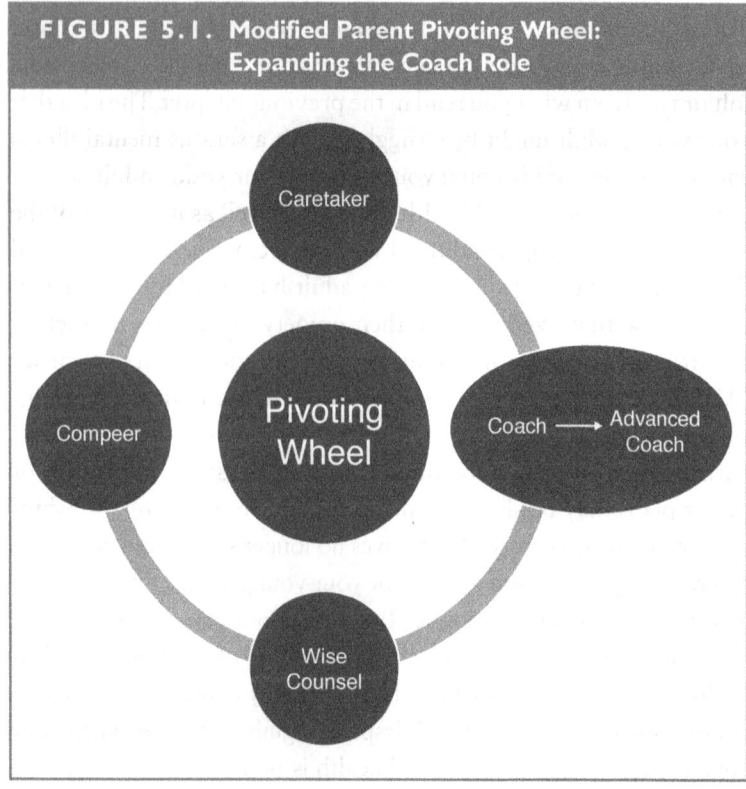

FIGURE 5.1. Modified Parent Pivoting Wheel: Expanding the Coach Role

to help parents deal with their adult child's more serious mental health issues. We want to make clear that these skills are useful for all parents and adding them to your tote bag is like having a good insurance policy for when you might need it down the road. Before we move into these new skills, however, let's discuss what you don't want to do as an advanced coach.

AVOID PERPETUAL CARETAKING OR DISENGAGING

The natural inclination for most parents of young adults with serious mental health issues is to pivot immediately from coach or advanced coach to caretaker. And in some situations, that pivot is appropriate. However, too often, parents will take up residence in the caretaker role and refuse to leave. Some parents may even waffle between returning to caretaker and detaching from the situation altogether. The sense of being overwhelmed competes with their concern for their young adults and, at least momentarily, they seek escape. When a parent waffles or tries to escape, it can be helpful for them to take a beat, notice their desire to escape, and give themselves permission to feel that temporarily. This feeling is understandable given the level of stress they are experiencing. In some instances, family history may get in the way of your being able to effectively handle what is happening with your adult child. In either case, it is important to realize that such tactics block one's ability to grow as a person and a parent.

Determining when it is appropriate to be in the caretaker role is critical. In addition to assessing your young adult's levels of distress and functioning, you must also pay attention to signs of whether a crisis is brewing. For example, if they are making statements about hopelessness for the future, feeling worthless, or wanting to harm themselves or others, engaging in high-risk behaviors (e.g., reckless driving, overusing substances, self-injury such as cutting), you need to step in to ensure their safety. This is part of the caretaker role.

EXHIBIT 5.1. Advanced Coaching Skills

- Educate yourself about your young adult's mental health issue (see Chapter 4).
- Reframe your thoughts.
- Recognize and address collateral damage.
- Seek support from others.

However, in the absence of such crisis situations, taking up residence in the caretaker role is counterproductive to the well-being of you and your young adult. Keep in mind, you spent many years as a caretaker, and you might feel very comfortable being back in that role. What is optimal here, however, is for the parent of a newly diagnosed adult child or one in the aftermath of a mental health crisis to act as a caretaker at times but to be wary of remaining in this role for a prolonged period. Remember, as a perpetual caretaker, you remain in the "doing for" mode, which takes away your young adult's self-confidence and autonomy. Developmental tasks in the emerging adult stage are all about exploring identity, relationships, career possibilities, and finding their own purpose and meaning for their lives. When you get in the way of their efforts in any of these areas, you undermine their ability in the future to become independent and autonomous adults. Essentially, there is the danger of them becoming *developmentally frozen*.

You already know how important it is to educate yourself about your young adult's mental health issue. Let's turn now to other skills you will use as an advanced coach (see Exhibit 5.1).

REFRAME YOUR THOUGHTS

In Chapter 2, we stressed the significance of attending to your feelings and learning how to manage them more effectively. Now in your role as advanced coach, we encourage you to get a handle on how your thoughts may be irrational at times and interfere with your effectiveness with your young adult. Cognitive behavioral psychologists believe that our thoughts are powerful determinants of our emotions and actions; essentially, it is our thinking that drives the bus. These psychologists specialize in helping people identify their thoughts, explore their impact, and assess their usefulness. They also teach skills for how to replace unhelpful thoughts with more balanced ones. Cognitive behavior therapy (CBT) allows you to change your perspective and regulate your own emotions so that you can attend to what is happening without overreacting.

We all have a constant stream of thoughts running through our minds every day, and it is overwhelming to imagine paying attention to all of these. The ones that are most memorable, and keep repeating in our heads, we refer to as *self-talk*. Our self-talk can be both a blessing and a curse. For example, positive self-talk—"You can do it, you've got this, don't give up"—can motivate us to persevere when things are rough. On the other hand, self-talk can work against us when it is inaccurate, negative, or critical. For example, telling yourself "You messed up, you are a loser, you will never succeed" works against your ability to stay the course when the going gets tough.

The reality is that many of our thoughts are just plain false. Psychologists have, for example, identified more than 20 types of thinking errors (Boyes, 2013). The bulk of these is characterized by our tendency to lean into the negative thoughts and to minimize the positive ones. You have likely heard the idea that our negative thoughts hold on like Velcro and our positive thoughts seem to slip away like sliding off Teflon. The tendency to think negatively (negativity bias) is natural for all of us because it served an important survival function for our ancestors who lived with daily life and death situations. Unfortunately, the tendency to focus on negative experiences and feedback and ignore more positive events and feedback remained with us long after the life-and-death scenarios disappeared from our daily lives. Once in a while, however, our negative thoughts do accurately reflect reality. In such cases, the brain sends us into flight-or-fight mode and, in so doing, ensures our survival!

Most of the time, however, holding on to negative thinking limits us in terms of opportunities and relationships, not to mention our ability to see the upside to our lives. For example, imagine that you are up for a promotion at work. Your supervisor brings you in for your performance review and overall gives you high ratings for your work. She mentions two areas in which she believes you need to improve and suggests ways you might go about this. She concludes the review by saying you are doing a commendable job and encourages you to keep up the good work. Of the 20 or so performance areas, only two are negative. However, you zero in on the two areas you need to improve and forget all the positive comments your supervisor shared with you. Your emphasis on what you did "wrong" overshadows the many qualities that make you a good employee.

This is similar to glass-half-full versus glass-half-empty thinking. We all know folks who approach life with a glass-half-full mindset. They are able to see the upside of a situation or a person and move forward into their day. We also know folks who take a glass-half-empty view of life. They live with a sense of not having enough and not being enough because there is more that they should be, know, or possess. They apply this to others as well. So instead of seeing their young adult as a "work in progress" growing toward adulthood, they see only the shortcomings and the areas in which they are lacking. Some folks will tell you that this prevents them from being disappointed. Sadly, however, they never get to experience the goodness that exists in their lives every day. The ability to see your young adult from the work in progress perspective is essential. Exhibit 5.2 provides an exercise to help you when you feel yourself slipping into a negativity spiral.

EXHIBIT 5.2. When You Feel Yourself Sinking Into Negativity

- STOP.
- Take a breath.
- Name three things that are going well for you today.

Before you can reframe your thoughts, it's important to understand the kinds of cognitive errors we are all prone to making. In Table 5.1, we identify those cognitive errors that are common among parents of young adults with mental health disorders. For example, when you engage in catastrophizing about your young adult's mental health issue by thinking that your child "will never be able to have a successful career or a stable relationship," this will block your ability to respond appropriately. Simply put, reframing your thoughts is a process of recognizing when your thinking is off kilter in a given situation and that you need to reset it using a different perspective. This means you replace an irrational thought with one that is more in tune with reality. So in this instance, a parent might say, "My child might struggle a bit, but they can still have a successful career."

Reframing your thoughts can serve as an effective go-to coping strategy during times of emotional distress. To make the process more user-friendly, we would like to provide a step-by-step set of instructions to assist you in reframing your thoughts (Exhibit 5.3). Creating a new perspective through reframing your thoughts will offer you some sense of control with a feeling of calm and ultimately your distress will begin to diminish.

Using Exhibit 5.3, let's take a closer look at how reframing your thoughts can help lower your stress and raise your ability to communicate with your young adult. For Arturo, catastrophizing about his son's future does little to calm him down or help him talk with his

143

TABLE 5.1. Cognitive Errors

Error	Example
Catastrophizing: Thinking the WORST	Arturo tells himself that since his son is "dropping out" of school he is going to end up on the streets without a job. He will never go anywhere.
Overgeneralization: Believing that what happened in one situation will repeat itself in similar situations	Lucia contacts the university to find out about a medical leave of absence. Arturo tells himself if Daniel quits school, he will be a quitter for the rest of his life.
Should: Holding rigid expectations of self and others	Arturo tells himself that Daniel should not be in bed at 11:00 am. He should be out looking for a job.
Personalization: Believing that other people's behaviors, choices or reactions are directed at or about oneself	Arturo believes Daniel's staying in bed is a direct attack on him as a father and has nothing to do with being depressed.
Change fallacies: Believing the other person will change if you apply enough pressure	Arturo believes that if he keeps pressuring Daniel to change his behavior and get a job, good hard work will cure what's ailing him.
All-or-nothing thinking: Thinking in terms of extremes: good or bad, black or white, yes or no	Arturo fumes, "Either he gets a job this week or he has to move out!"

EXHIBIT 5.3. How to Reframe Your Thoughts

- NOTICE your thought.
- Take a breath and a few seconds to reflect.
- Challenge your thought with questions such as the following: Is this thought true? Is this thought helpful to me? Do I have evidence to support this thought? Am I confusing my thought with a fact?
- Replace your thought with a new, accurate, and more positive thought.

---

son. Instead, Arturo might try taking a moment and asking himself, "Where is the evidence for this?" As Arturo reflects on this question, he quickly realizes that Daniel has done pretty well so far with his academics and his baseball. "That kid's got grit! Maybe things aren't so bad with him." By tuning in to what's working in Daniel's life, he can reframe his thoughts as follows: "My son is having a rough time right now. This doesn't mean he is stuck there forever." Such a reframe allows Arturo to view the situation as temporary, rather than something that will never change. This gives him hope for the future.

Another cognitive error that parents tend to have is overgeneralizing their young adult's current situation to their entire future. When Lucia arranges a medical leave of absence for Daniel, Arturo sees this as quitting and thinks his son will always be a quitter. Again, Arturo takes a moment and considers the evidence. Daniel has not been a quitter in the past. Even with his ADHD, he has managed to keep going. This frees Arturo up to reframe this thought: "A leave of absence will give Daniel the time to get himself together so he can return to school."

As parents, we are all guilty of the "shoulds" from time to time. In this case, Arturo thinks Daniel "should" be out of bed and job hunting. "After all, everyone I know who is successful gets up and going by 6:00 a.m. I always do, and so did my father." Reframing involves challenging this belief in light of the current situation, where Daniel's depression plays a part in his sleeping patterns. Arturo needs to be able to empathize with his son and understand his struggle. "I need to cut him some slack. He can apply for a job online or head out later in the day."

When we personalize our young adult's behavior as somehow a reflection on us, we stop seeing their behavior from an objective point of view. Arturo thinks that Daniel's isolating himself in his room is a means of avoiding him. Instead of feeling sorry for himself or angry with Daniel, Arturo might reframe his thoughts and convey some understanding of what's happening with his son. "I'm upset by Daniel's behavior, and yet I know his isolation is about his depression and not about me."

Change fallacies trick many of us into believing that if we just push harder, we can make our young adults do what we think is best. Does this sound familiar? Arturo believes if he just keeps nagging his son, Daniel will hop out of bed and get a job. Good luck with that, right? A reframe that might be helpful here is for Arturo first to realize that no matter how hard he pushes, Daniel is not able to respond. Due to his depression, he lacks the energy and motivation right now to look for work. Arturo might say to himself, "While I want to push him out of bed, that's not going to happen. I need to be patient here."

When we are stressed, we can easily slip into seeing the world in all-or-nothing terms. Arturo is no different. He masks his fear about his son with anger and makes the threat of Daniel having to move out if he doesn't have work by the end of the week. After some deep breaths, perhaps he can see the fallacy of false threats and respond more appropriately. "I'm so angry that he's stuck in bed. But I have to tell myself kicking him out won't do any good. Where would he go? How would he pay for the rent? Sometimes

I get ahead of myself, and don't think clearly. I just want my son to be okay."

When we are distressed, we may act as if our thoughts are facts, often termed "cognitive fusion" (Hayes, 2005) without taking time to examine other alternatives. This is a basic premise of acceptance and commitment therapy, which is closely aligned with CBT. For example, Lucia thinks Arturo is selfish and uncaring in his relationship with his son. This thought leads her to be angry and resentful toward Arturo, and they end up avoiding each other. One useful way for her to begin the process of exploring alternative perspectives about Arturo is to ask herself how useful her thinking is in getting her what she wants and values. In this case, what she really wants is for them to be able to communicate with and support each other in learning how to be better parents to Daniel. This allows her to see that this thought is not getting her where she wants to be. Rather than her thought being an absolute fact, she realizes that it may not be accurate at all. The caveat not to believe everything you think would be helpful to Lucia here. It will bolster both her and your ability to function effectively as an advanced coach.

ADDRESS COLLATERAL DAMAGE

Collateral damage is what happens to other family members when a young adult is in psychological distress. This involves recognizing the impact on each family member. Let's listen as Claire tells her story about a memorable incident that occurred shortly before Anne was hospitalized and diagnosed with bipolar disorder:

> It was a warm, relaxing July night when the sharp ring of my phone broke the stillness. I saw my sister's number on the screen and instantly tensed. Something was wrong. I knew it—

it was late and my sister lives in an even later time zone. I snatched up my phone.

"Laura, what is it?"

"It's Anne," her words tumbled out in an unsteady voice. "I just hung up with her. She told me she's leaving for Egypt in 2 days, and she doesn't want you and Stan to know. She begged me to promise not to tell you. She said if I did, she'd never speak to me again!"

Laura paused to catch her breath, and then continued, "Anne plans to leave a note for you saying she is on vacation and asking you not to notify the police that she was missing. I feel trapped between a rock and a hard place, but I had to let you know!"

I sat there totally stunned. Laura and I ended our call a few minutes later, and I turned to look at Stan who had overheard. We stared at each other, speechless. Who was this young woman? What planet did she come from? This was not our Anne, the girl we had raised.

Soon afterward, Anne stomped into the house slamming the door. She refused to look at us.

"We know about the trip," I said. "We're not happy about it, but we won't stop you. Please, Anne, leave us your itinerary, and make contact with us while you're away. We just want to know you're safe." My words were met with an icy silence.

The next day, I went to Anne's room and calmly asked if we could talk about what was happening. Anne flew into a rage, screaming and cursing at me in a torrent of verbal abuse. This was too much! I began to cry, and that is when Anne physically attacked me, pounding on my left arm as I tried to fend her off. Stan came running at the sound of the screaming and pulled Anne off of me. I sank to the floor sobbing while Anne bolted out of the room and down the stairs.

Anne grabbed her younger sister, flew out the front door, and we heard the roar of her car as she took off. Even though we said we were not going to prevent her from going on her trip, Anne impulsively went out and bought an old beat-up car to make her "escape." She was certain we would take the keys to the car she already had and keep her from leaving the next day.

Anne did indeed drive her "new" old clunker away with her suitcase packed the following morning. For the next 2 weeks, we heard nothing from her. She refused all contact with us, no calls, no texts, nothing. Those were two of the most gut-wrenching weeks of my life. My mind went into overdrive catastrophizing. "What-ifs" sent my anxiety through the roof. At the same time, the physical reminders of what Anne had done were clearly visible. My left arm was totally black and blue from the beating. I kept it hidden under a long sleeve shirt, not willing to explain the bruising to anyone. How could I tell my friends and coworkers that my daughter had done this to me?

All I knew was that my 19-year-old daughter was traveling somewhere in the world, and I had no clue where she was. Stan and I were in shock. Anne's sister, Sara, was scared for her sister and confused about why all this was happening. My sister felt guilty for betraying Anne's confidence but knew she had done the right thing in telling us what was going on. Meanwhile, I wondered what was happening to our family.

The struggle in Claire's family to come to terms with Anne's behavior is part of collateral damage. Claire's situation is not unlike other families whose young adults begin to show signs of mental illness. Her story underscores the chaotic and unpredictable world that can unfold inside the families of many emerging adults, especially when more serious mental illness appears. Learning to recognize and address collateral damage is another essential skill for an advanced coach. Let's return to Claire's story and consider the perspective of Sara, Anne's younger sister:

How does all this affect me? It's hard to deal with sometimes. As little kids Anne and I got along well. When we moved on to junior high though, things started to change. I always knew

Anne and I were very different from each other, and other people noticed it, too. Anne was quiet, very reserved; she would read all the time and loved to be alone. She also loved to take long hikes outdoors on the nature trails around where we lived. She was very smart and did well in school, especially in literature. I was the social butterfly and spent all my time outside of school involved in activities and being with my friends. I liked school, too, but I was good at different subjects than Anne; math and art were my favorite classes.

Anne went to college close to home and seemed to enjoy her new freedom and her classes. She was making friends and getting involved in various clubs and organizations on campus. I got to see her a good bit, even though she was living on campus. I noticed a rather sudden change in her midway through her freshman year. She became moody and irritable, much unlike the sister I had known, who had always been laid back and able to roll with whatever came her way. Mom and Dad and others around her noticed this as well.

The weird part was, she always dumped her anger on our parents; I never understood why. She rarely called them and almost never came home to visit. She complained to me that they were horrible parents, yet I could see nothing different in them or their behavior. She suddenly began contacting me and telling me things about her life but swore me to secrecy. I was never to tell Mom and Dad *anything* she told me. This was very upsetting to me. While it was nice to have some relationship with my sister, at the same time, I felt like I was walking on thin ice.

When Anne did come home on a weekend, everything had to go her way. If that didn't happen, she would scream awful things at Mom and Dad and storm out of the house and be gone sometimes for hours. When she finally did return, I never knew if there would be another explosion or if she would act like nothing had happened. Even though Anne was okay around me, I could see the stress she was causing our parents. The house reeked with tension. We could never tell when the next outburst would come. It wasn't a fun way to live. I decided the best thing for me was to go my own way and stay away from her. I focused on school and my friends, and I made sure not to do anything that would upset Mom and Dad. I felt so badly for them. Even when Anne was not at home, her anger and temper tantrums were never really gone from our home. It was awful and I couldn't fix it.

Sara, like many siblings, seems to take a backseat in the chaos that often swirls in the families of emerging adults who have mental health issues. Like Sara, Daniel's sister, Elena, appears to cope with the family's stress by staying under the radar. Much to her mother's frustration, Elena physically escapes the stress associated with Daniel's illness by spending all her time at a friend's home. In Sara's case, this means compensating for her sister's dysfunction by excelling in academics and seeking approval from her peers. She works to lessen the chaos and conflict in the household by keeping "secrets." This is not uncommon; some siblings act as mediators within their family unit in response to the tension and conflict among family members. Some siblings, like Sara, cope with feelings of powerlessness and a lack of control in the family, by striving to never rock the boat, by being "perfect," which may come at the cost of never being themselves. They might further assume a caretaking role for their emotionally troubled friends and others outside the family.

Siblings of young adults with anxiety, depression, and other related symptoms often report feeling abandoned, invisible, or forgotten by their parents. In many cases siblings may be asked to assume more household responsibilities and even take care of their sibling with a mental health disorder. These responsibilities can have both positive and negative consequences. For some siblings, this experience is connected to personal loss of freedom and an increase in stress. It may also lead to feelings of resentment. For others, such a responsibility helps to foster their own maturity and personal growth as well as to contribute to family unity and functioning. Some siblings experience significant pressure, either self-imposed or from parents, as a result of trying to compensate for the ill sibling. Still others may work to conceal or minimize their own problems so as not to give their parents any cause to worry.

It is also common for siblings to experience anxiety and a fear of becoming mentally ill themselves. This may be especially true in cases where their siblings have disorders that are known to have a higher likelihood of being inherited. Many siblings are apt to experience survivor guilt, which refers to sadness and remorse associated with living after a destructive traumatic event (e.g., mass shooting, hurricane, airplane crash) when others lost their lives or their lives as they knew them. In this case, the traumatic event is a sibling's mental health disorder. Some siblings also feel a sense of guilt either for failing to support their ill sibling or for failing to recognize their symptoms before a formal diagnosis.

In many families, a culture of secrecy exists when an adult child is diagnosed with a mental health disorder. This may come in the form of a directive from one or both parents not to share information about what was happening with anyone else outside the family. However, it is clear that siblings need a forum for dealing with their feelings. Many well siblings, for example, internalize or negate their feelings. A common belief is that not talking about something prevents it from being painful.

When a discussion is opened, parents need to be attentive to the ways in which they communicate with all their children about mental illnesses. This helps to minimize the risks associated with the surrounding social stigma. Children should be invited to ask questions and identify their feelings. It is also necessary for parents to pursue shared family activities and traditions to maintain a sense of stability.

Unfortunately, in our clinical work, we have found most families err on the side of not communicating enough about difficult and emotionally painful issues. We have also discovered that parents are afraid of talking about such issues for fear that by doing so, they may make the feelings grow more intense and difficult to manage.

Many families struggle to cope in silence; some of this is due to the negative beliefs, stigma, and shame that continues to shroud mental illness. It keeps them from being open with others for fear that they will be judged as bad parents. Parents may also feel guarded about talking with a friend regarding their adult child's mental health issues because the friend's young adult appears to have launched into adulthood and is doing well.

Many parents share the concern and frustration Lucia feels as she struggles to help Daniel. Much like Claire, Lucia is used to stepping in and doing all she can to make sure Daniel's needs are met, but now that won't work. She likely feels more and more helpless each time Daniel fails to follow through. For example, Daniel says he will talk to the admissions office at the community college about taking some classes but never does. Lucia is at her wits' end.

SEEK SUPPORT FROM OTHERS

This brings us to the final advanced coaching skill that we introduced at the beginning of the chapter: seek support from others. We see support-seeking as a two-pronged process. First is the informational prong, where parents might seek support from other parents who share their challenges or professionals who help parents with these challenges. Consider participating in online and in-person educational and support groups. One particularly helpful program is the National Alliance for the Mentally Ill's Family-to-Family program, a free, eight-session educational program for family members. Many of the national organizations listed in Exhibit 5.4 also provide contact information on support groups for parents at the state and local levels. Equipped with this kind of objective information, parents are better able to understand their adult child's mental health disorder.

> **EXHIBIT 5.4. Self-Help Resources for Parents**
>
> - Depression and Bipolar Support Alliance (https://www.dbsalliance. org/). Offers online and print resources, in-person and online support groups for mood disorders, including depression and bipolar disorder.
> - Families for Depression Awareness (https://www.familyaware.org/). Provides families of people living with mood disorders, including depression or bipolar disorder, with education and support.
> - National Alliance for the Mentally Ill's (NAMI) Family Support Group (https://www.nami.org/). A peer-led, structured, and free support group for adults with loved ones who have symptoms of a mental health issue.
> - Mental Health America's Family Support Network (https://mhanational. org/parent-support-network). A facilitated, free support group (virtual and in-person) for parents of children, ages 1 to 25, who have mental health challenges.

Once they have this understanding, they can more effectively engage in difficult dialogues with their young adult.

The second prong has to do with the emotional benefits of seeking support, the realization that you are not alone in your struggle. There are others out there who are looking for suggestions of how to better navigate the turbulent waters and maintain their own well-being and sanity. Sharing the struggles, the joys, the frustrations with others who are on a similar journey can help you to feel understood and less isolated. You begin to realize that mental illness is much more common than you might have thought, and the stigma you feel surrounding mental health issues begins to fade. You may choose to get into therapy for yourself, which is also a way of finding much-needed support.

One caveat as you seek out support: All groups and all therapists are not equal! It is important to find a group or a therapist that will meet your needs and support your growth in a positive direction. As therapists we know from experience that people need to trust their gut. If the therapist or group does not offer a constructive environment in which to share your feelings and concerns and does not fuel your growth, then it's time to look for alternative sources of support.

SUMMARY

Whew! This is a lot of information to absorb. The distress associated with mental illness in adult children reverberates throughout the entire family. When your adult child is newly diagnosed, in the early phases of treatment, or in the midst of a mental health crisis, you may likely need to expand your repertoire of coaching skills by learning how to minimize your own distress and the tendency to catastrophize. It is also necessary to equip yourself with the comprehensive knowledge about mental health issues and address possible collateral damage in your family.

In the next chapter, we present important information for you about resources for treatment and strategies for communicating with your adult child about treatment options. We enumerate current challenges you as a mental health consumer and your family experience in dealing with the mental health system. The challenges emerging adults may face as they navigate the health care systems for the first time as legal adults can be daunting.

POINTS TO POCKET

- Remember: Negative thinking is our default mode. We need to challenge the accuracy of what we tell ourselves.
- You are not your thoughts—but you can use your thoughts to create a more positive mindset.

- Ernest Hemingway (1929) wrote, "You are so brave and quiet, I forgot you are suffering" (p. 69). As a parent, be sure to be aware of the effect of your young adult's mental health issues on other family members.

- Breaking the silence about mental health disorders, even in our own families, is imperative. To borrow Glenn Close's (2010) phrase, we need "more sunlight, candor, unashamed conversation" (para. 13) around mental health issues.

- As a parent of a young adult with a mental health concern, it is okay to have bad days, and it is also okay to ask for help and support when you need it. In fact, this is an essential part of taking care of yourself as you continue your journey.

CHAPTER 6

HELP! I NEED SOMEBODY, NOT JUST ANYBODY

Be strong enough to stand alone, smart enough to know when you need help, and brave enough to ask for it.
—Ziad K. Abdelnour, *Economic Warfare*

If your young adult has a serious mental health issue, you are in a unique position to be a trusted advisor to them as they begin to navigate the complicated and challenging road of the mental health care system. To carry out this important task, you must first understand that system yourself. Our purpose in this chapter is to equip you with additional skills to enhance your coach role as you talk with your adult child about treatment. The idea that your young adult needs mental health treatment can feel overwhelming and frightening for you as the parent. It is likely equally disheartening for your young adult, yet still, they will be the one making the decisions. Remember, moms and dads, you are not in the driver's seat. It is up to your young adult to make decisions regarding their treatment. This is especially challenging for many parents because emerging adults, in general, are reluctant to seek mental health care. We know that early intervention contributes to more positive outcomes. When a young adult refuses or is ambivalent about treatment, their situation may worsen. The stories of parents who watch from the sidelines while their young adult's symptoms spiral out of control into a crisis are heartbreaking.

We begin with an overview of treatment options (talk therapy, medication, expressive therapies, and exercise) as well as a list of types of treatment providers working in the field of mental health.

We hope to deepen your understanding of how to navigate this stressful and possibly unfamiliar territory. And, of course, we offer some additional skills that are necessary when your young adult is in psychological distress or has a serious mental health disorder.

NAVIGATING THE MAZE

As a parent of a young adult with mental illness, you may find the process of locating a mental health provider to be much like the experience of walking through a maze. Our current mental health care system is in deep trouble. Provider shortages are especially acute in rural areas and in some stressed cities throughout the United States. The waiting list for providers, particularly psychiatrists, can be months long in some geographic areas. The United States already had a shortage of psychiatrists before the COVID pandemic. Unfortunately, the pandemic triggered a significant increase in psychological distress including mental health disorders among adults. At present, there are far more people in need of psychiatrists than there are available psychiatrists.

Providers across clinics and practice settings often don't coordinate care and treatment planning, leaving the door open for working at cross purposes with one another. Despite the high incidence of addiction found with mood and anxiety disorders, substance abuse and mental health are often treated as separate entities, where their practitioners seldom coordinate care. As noted in Chapter 4, many mental health disorders are periodic and urgent and, if untreated, can result in a crisis that is life-threatening.

For those emerging adults attending universities, counseling centers face a soaring demand for services. At the same time, the number of staff remains the same (Center for Collegiate Mental Health, 2022). In addition, university counseling centers are experiencing considerable staff turnover and the impact on remaining staff includes low morale, higher caseloads and overall workload, burnout, loss of trust in leadership, exhaustion and fatigue, etc. (Gorman et al., 2020). Students seeking mental health services are often put on waiting lists, given a limit on the number of therapy sessions they are allotted per semester or year, or are referred out to a community mental health agency or private practice. In recent years, a small percentage of university counseling centers have begun charging students' private insurance for the provision of services. This is often problematic when the young adult wants to keep their treatment a secret, and the bill and explanation of services is mailed to the parents.

Your experience of finding effective mental health treatment can leave you feeling as though you are in the maze, going in circles, and getting nowhere. This is a great time to remember to breathe. Throughout this chapter, we provide information you will need along this journey; some of it may feel overwhelming at times. To better prepare you for any dead ends along the way, we identify a variety of potential difficulties you may experience in your attempts to locate professional help for your young adult. It is important to remember that perseverance and patience are essential tools as you navigate through the mental health care system. Please bear in mind, though, that despite its complexity, a maze does have a path through it. Take heart, parents, your persistence and patience will pay off.

FINDING HELP FOR YOUR YOUNG ADULT

Consider the following: Most people invest far more time and energy in selecting a computer or flat screen television than they do choosing a mental health care provider. Most read about the newest technology, peruse online reviews, consult with friends and family, and ask lots of questions before investing in technologically oriented devices. Decisions about mental health care are comparatively short-changed. Does this make any sense? In this section, we present a brief overview of the mental health care system with tips for navigating the maze. This is the first step of educating yourself about the treatment process and an essential component to carry in your tote bag.

The Importance of Finding a Specialist

The task of finding an effective mental health provider for your adult child is likely to be confusing and overwhelming. For those who have insurance, it is not always easy to identify providers who are accepting new patients. If your young adult is still under your insurance, you may need to clarify what your mental health benefits are and which providers are covered under your insurance plan. Even if your adult child's options are limited by your insurance, it is still important that you research the credentials of each of the providers covered on your plan. In addition, it is often unclear what your total out-of-pocket costs will be.

In many instances, parents and their adult children instinctively turn to their primary care provider or general physician for help with anxiety, depression, and other forms of emotional distress. Most general practitioners will prescribe antidepressants and antianxiety medications and provide a list of mental health referrals, websites, other informational resources, and crisis resources. Approximately 80% of antidepressant and antianxiety medications are prescribed by primary care providers (Insel, 2022). Your primary care provider can determine whether your young adult's behaviors or symptoms are suggestive of a physical or medical problem such as thyroid disease, Lyme disease, neuroendocrine tumors, and others, but not a mental health disorder. However, this provider, in most cases, does not have the specialized knowledge, training, and experience that a psychiatrist or mental health care provider has to diagnose and treat mental illness.

We use an analogy here: If you break your arm, you see an orthopedist; if you have symptoms of a mental illness, we encourage you to see a psychiatrist. Although both your general practitioner and a psychiatrist are medical doctors, only the psychiatrist is trained to evaluate, diagnose, and treat mental illness. Because there are no tests available to confirm suspected diagnoses of mental health disorders as there are with physical illnesses, we encourage you to consult with a psychiatrist.

In Chapter 4, we underscored the formidable challenges associated with making an accurate diagnosis of anxiety, depression, bipolar, and other related disorders as well as the imperative for doing this in a timely fashion. These situations demand a high level of expertise. As you will soon discover, prescribing the medications used to treat more severe anxiety, depression, and bipolar disorder also requires an advanced level of proficiency. It is important to note that most psychiatrists do not provide talk therapy. This makes it necessary to engage the services of another mental health provider, one who offers talk therapy or counseling. Most people wind up having two providers, a psychiatrist and a talk therapist. We absolutely recommend this. Please note that in some states, psychologists, with additional training, are able to prescribe certain medications to treat mental health disorders. We say this to alleviate possible confusion should you live in one of these states.

The Importance of Having an Assessment

In Chapter 3, we described the complications that can arise when your young adult is engaged in unhealthy behaviors (e.g., substance and internet misuse, unhealthy eating and excessive exercising) as a means of coping with their psychological distress. In many cases, these coping behaviors can develop into substance use disorders and/or eating disorders. For this reason, it is imperative that a qualified mental health professional complete a comprehensive assessment and consider the need for a referral to a mental health specialist who works with substance issues or eating concerns. Typically, addictions and eating disorders specialists are certified through additional coursework and other requirements.

We recommend that parents and emerging adults consider obtaining a neuropsychological assessment when there is reason to suspect a neurodevelopmental disorder (e.g., attention-deficit/hyperactivity disorder [ADHD], a specific learning disorder). A neuropsychologist is the most qualified provider to diagnose neurodevelopmental disorders. They are trained to administer and interpret a comprehensive variety of specialized tests to help diagnose disorders and to guide practitioners in treatment planning.

The purpose of the assessment is to identify your young adult's cognitive strengths and weaknesses and to describe their emotional, social, and behavioral functioning. For treatment to be effective, an accurate diagnosis is essential. All too often, it seems neurodevelopmental disorders such as ADHD are diagnosed following completion of some brief self-report questionnaires. Such questionnaires cannot be considered an assessment, making the results questionable. Although the costs associated with these evaluations are often intimidating, the test results are extremely helpful when the diagnosis is in question.

It is essential to understand the importance of a comprehensive evidence-based treatment approach, which includes talk therapy as well as medication. As we discuss later in this chapter, it is also important to consider the use of adjuncts to treatment, such as exercise and expressive therapies, for use with emerging adults.

Who Can Prescribe Medications, and Who Can Provide Talk Therapy?

The process of seeking talk therapy begins with consideration of which type of provider is appropriate to work with your emerging adult. There are multiple types of practitioners with various credentials and specialties. The professional boards for each state evaluate all applications for licensure and issue licenses to those professionals who qualify. Each board establishes rules and regulations to ensure the competence and integrity of its providers.

Even if your insurance requires you to use in-network providers and your options are limited, it is vital that you understand the level of training and credentials of your providers. See Table 6.1 for a list of the types of mental health practitioners.

Most psychiatrists limit their practices to assessment and medication management, rather than talk therapy. Psychiatrists are required to complete 4 years of medical school and a residency program (3–7 years of clinical training). They are the most extensively trained of all psychiatric providers. Other options for medication provision and management include physician assistants (PAs), psychiatric or mental health nurse practitioners, and some psychologists.

TABLE 6.1. Mental Health Providers

Qualification	Providers
Can prescribe medications	Psychiatrists Physician's assistants Psychiatric or mental health nurse practitioners Qualifying psychologists in some states
Can provide talk therapy	Psychologists Licensed professional counselors/licensed mental health counselors Licensed clinical social workers Licensed marriage and family therapists

To become a physician assistant, a person must earn a bachelor's degree in a relevant field and graduate from a master's PA program. All PAs are required to have some level of physician supervision regardless of where they live.

There are currently approximately 22 states that grant full authority to psychiatric or mental health nurse practitioners (PMHNPs) to prescribe medications without the supervision of a physician. The PMHNP typically completes an undergraduate degree in nursing and a master of science in nursing (MSN) degree (or also a doctor of nursing practice degree), which generally takes a minimum of 2 years.

At present, a handful of states (i.e., New Mexico, Louisiana, Illinois, Iowa, and Idaho) have provisions under law for qualifying, specially trained psychologists to prescribe psychotropic medication. In addition to the doctoral degree, prescribing psychologists in these states are required to complete the equivalent of a master's degree in psychopharmacology plus an extensive supervised clinical rotation in psychopharmacology.

In addition to those providers who prescribe medications, there are a number of other options for your adult child for talk therapy. Psychologists have the most extensive graduate training and are required to complete a doctorate in clinical or counseling psychology which can take 4 to 6 years of coursework and a full year of internship. Psychologists are also trained to provide psychological testing. Licensed professional counselors (LPCs)/licensed mental health counselors (LMHCs) and licensed clinical social workers (LCSWs) have a master's degree and (usually) advanced training in psychotherapy (i.e., practicum and internship). LCSWs typically have special expertise in navigating the social services system and can often serve as case managers. Licensed marriage and family therapists (LMFTs) have a master's degree and are trained primarily to provide couples/marital and family counseling. However, with special training, all of these practitioners can provide group, family, and couples/marital therapy as well. In addition, it is important to note that some of these master's-level professionals have taken additional training to become certified in substance abuse counseling.

Finding Providers

Many mental health practitioners promote themselves through online postings that include a photograph, a short professional biography typically including information about credentials, and a description of their approach to therapy, clinical interests, fees and/or which insurances they accept. Psychology Today (https://www.psychologytoday.com/us/therapists) is perhaps the most popular website for anyone looking for a mental health professional. This excellent resource allows you to search by specialty, location, insurance coverage, and more.

As you review the list of providers, please consider each professional's depth of clinical experience, both in terms of working specifically with young adults and with anxiety, depression, bipolar, and other related disorders. Not all providers have the specialized knowledge and years of experience to work with the unique population of today's young adults. For example, in Chapter 3, we discussed what can happen when your young adult is anxious, depressed, or otherwise psychologically distressed and begins to engage in substance misuse, unhealthy eating, internet misuse, and other risky behaviors, including self-injury. When these behaviors accompany mental health issues, diagnosis and treatment can be especially challenging.

At a minimum, your selection of possible providers should encompass those who are licensed in the state where your emerging adult resides. To be licensed in a state, all applicants' education and training must meet the professional standards of their specific discipline, and they must pass the licensure exam. This offers some comfort relative to competence. You can check your state's licensing board website to find the licensure status of any mental health professional. Each state's licensing board will also provide information to consumers about any validated ethics complaints against providers.

Understand HIPAA

The federal Health Insurance Portability and Accountability Act (HIPAA) was created in 1996 to protect patients' medical records, identifying patient information, health insurance information, and other data. This law provides legal adults with the right to access their medical records, request a copy of their records, and control who may view their medical information. The bottom line is that HIPAA prevents your young adult's medical records from being shared without their permission or from being taken advantage of in some way.

Because your young adult is at least 18 years of age, they can legally make decisions regarding their medical records; they decide with whom their records can be shared. This might be unsettling to you as a parent. However, there are times when exceptions to HIPAA are made, and medical records can be shared. For example, the HIPAA law contains a provision related to inpatient substance and mental health treatment that permits hospital personnel to disclose health care information in the case of an emergency. Such emergencies include a young adult threatening to harm themselves or others, or one who is incapacitated and whose emergency contact information cannot be found. This also includes a young adult with a communicable disease who has come in contact with others. In these cases, health care providers are permitted to use professional judgment to reach out to parents or advocates and let them know the location and condition of their young adult. Only the amount of information necessary to manage the situation should be shared. Parents sometimes report frustration with mental health providers who seem reluctant to disclose information to them regarding their young adult. Some providers may not clearly understand HIPAA's exceptions and others might believe that, in being overprotective, they are doing what is best for their young adult clients.

It is important for you as parents to know that HIPAA allows you to provide information to the treatment provider about your young adult when they cannot communicate for themselves, such as when they are in a manic or psychotic state. You can also provide information in instances when you have a compelling reason to believe your young adult has not shared important details about their situation. The treatment provider can listen to all you have to say without violating HIPAA, but it is unlikely they will share anything with you.

If your young adult is enrolled at a college or university, sharing and receiving information about them will likely be easier than if they are in the workforce. At college counseling centers, HIPAA does not limit the ability of families to reach out to treatment providers, but parents frequently lack this awareness. Parents are legally permitted to share concerns with and provide information about their young adult to a college counselor or student affairs personnel. Information you may choose to share includes past successful or unsuccessful treatment experiences, current medical conditions, special needs, and so on. It's important to keep in mind that communication is one-way unless your adult child has given their counselor permission to share relevant treatment information with you. The counselor then always has the right to decide whether to share any of your communication with their young adult client. They will base their decision on what they believe is in the best interest of their client. Keep in mind that residence hall directors, the dean of students, and other university administrators, unlike counselors, are not bound by confidentiality and are free to share information with you if they so choose.

Both college students and those young adults in the workforce can decide what information they would like shared with parents or others they may designate through the use of a medical power of attorney or a release of information. Many families hold discussions about access to health information, particularly physical and medical issues. We recommend having similar discussions regarding mental health information. Emerging adults who are already receiving mental health counseling should be encouraged by parents to consider signing authorization forms that would permit parents or family members to be informed of any changes in their adult child's mental health status.

TALK THERAPY TREATMENTS

Talk therapy, also known as psychotherapy, can be provided in many settings. Regardless of where it takes place, it should be evidence based, which means that the treatment procedures are well researched and documented over thousands of participants. Evidence-based practice in mental health care demands that therapeutic approaches and techniques be supported by such research. In addition to the signs and symptoms of mental illness, evidence-based practice requires therapists to consider the patient's culture, daily life realities, and values and preferences when making treatment recommendations. See Table 6.2 for a list of some of the many evidence-based psychotherapy approaches for use with generalized anxiety disorder, major depressive disorder, and bipolar disorder.

A word of caution: The bumper sticker from the '60s that commanded us to "question authority" is applicable now more than ever. If your young adult's provider is making recommendations that raise concerns for you, you can encourage your young adult to initiate a

TABLE 6.2. Examples of Evidence-Based Therapies

Disorder	Examples
Major Depressive Disorder	Cognitive behavioral analysis system Rational emotive behavioral therapy Short-term psychodynamic therapy Interpersonal psychotherapy Cognitive therapy Emotion focused therapy Acceptance and commitment therapy
Generalized Anxiety Disorder	Cognitive and behavioral therapy
Bipolar Disorder	Cognitive therapy Family focused therapy Interpersonal and social rhythm therapy Psychoeducation

conversation with the provider about their rationale and reasoning behind the treatment plan. Asking questions is always a good idea, particularly when you find yourself in unknown territory. And please keep in mind that not all the options are available in all locations.

So far, we have talked about what's known as outpatient therapy, which is by far the most common type of treatment for young adults in psychological distress. This involves seeing a mental health professional for talk therapy once or twice a week in a community clinic, private practice setting, or perhaps a university counseling center. Such treatment may also involve periodic visits with a medical provider qualified to dispense psychiatric medications. But two common alternative options are telehealth and hospital-based treatment.

Telehealth Mental Health Services

The COVID-19 pandemic has changed how and when people work. For example, some therapists only see patients in person, while others only use telehealth platforms (the use of videoconferencing technology such as Zoom or Vimeo to provide mental health services), and some offer a hybrid of the two. It is critically important for you and your emerging adult to think about what format would best meet their needs. Given the nature of anxiety, depression, bipolar disorder, and related disorders, together with the need for a strong therapeutic connection, we believe in-person sessions are optimal whenever possible. However, telehealth services can provide quality care. With the shortage of providers in many locations and many individuals' limited access to transportation, telehealth services are a viable alternative to face-to-face therapy sessions. Telehealth might also be a more natural fit for the more tech-savvy young adult. Plus, this option may provide more opportunities for your young adult to find services, particularly in more rural locations. Getting the necessary treatment is more important than how that treatment is delivered in most cases.

Hospital-Based Treatment

Hospital-based treatment, also called inpatient treatment, is used for situations in which the symptoms of mental health disorders are acute or your adult child's personal safety is in jeopardy. In these circumstances it is necessary to move to a more structured, safe space. Some inpatient settings specialize in specific issues, such as substance abuse or eating disorders.

Inpatient settings are highly structured and supervised. Patients are closely monitored to make sure they remain safe, and their daily activities consist of various supervised therapeutic activities, such as group therapy, individual therapy, and art therapy. Patients may stay for varying lengths of time depending on various factors, such as insurance benefits, availability of beds within the hospital setting, risk of self-harm or harm to others, the patient's specific diagnosis, and so on. This is an excellent option when a problem is particularly urgent, to the point where the individual is at risk of hurting themselves or others. However, the downside is that inpatient hospitalizations are expensive and restrict the freedoms that are so key to the developmental needs of emerging adults.

Let's return to Claire's situation from Chapter 4 where her daughter Anne is in crisis and her personal safety is clearly at risk, necessitating her involuntary hospitalization.

> After the call from the police that Anne had been picked up while wandering the streets aimlessly in an agitated state and had been hospitalized in the psych unit, I was terrified. The days that followed were a blur. Anne was heavily medicated and really out of it. There was a lot of back-and-forth with her psychiatrist, the social worker, and our insurance company about her treatment after her discharge from the hospital. For me, these were the worst days of my life. Finally, arrangements were made for Anne to participate in a partial hospitalization program. In this program, she was able to get treatment at the hospital 3 full days a week. Each evening, she came home, had dinner with us, and slept in her own bed. This semblance of normalcy was what saved me—and actually the whole family.

Anne's case illustrates how treatment options sometimes have to expand beyond weekly outpatient sessions to include more intensive treatment. It is important to note that inpatient treatment programs generally vary in intensity. Intensive outpatient programs provide the most comprehensive and time intensive treatment programs for persons who are newly discharged from hospital settings. Persons who have been diagnosed with mental health disorders are able to receive daily therapy and return home at night to sleep. Partial hospitalization programs, such as the one Anne was in, usually entail psychoeducation and therapy during the day, approximately three times per week. As Claire indicated, such types of treatment allow the family to retain some sense of normalcy while they and their young adult navigate the turbulence that has rocked their world.

👓 PSYCHOPHARMACOLOGICAL TREATMENTS

The terms *psychopharmacological* and *psychotropic* are used interchangeably to mean treatments involving medication for mental illnesses. Medication can often be a necessary component of treatment for mental health disorders. More and more adults of all ages are taking psychotropic medications without participating in psychotherapy (Terlizzi & Norris, 2021), despite research evidence that supports the effectiveness of combining talk therapy with medication (Barkham & Lambert, 2021). The choice to forgo psychotherapy may be due in part to the higher volume of patients being treated in primary care settings and the expenses associated with therapy. The practice of direct-to-consumer marketing of pharmaceuticals, including advertisements for psychotropic medications on television, in magazines, on websites, and on social media, is commonplace and often prompts patients to request these medications by name during office visits. On the plus side, this marketing helps educate the public and possibly aids in destigmatizing mental illness. However, these advertisements may lead to false perceptions that medications are magic pills that will allow a person to live happily ever after. Undoubtedly, you've listened to TV commercials for psychotropic medications that list the many possible side effects in 15 seconds flat. Additionally, the Food and Drug Administration (FDA) has issued a warning, specific to children, adolescents, and young adults for a number of antidepressants. Providers and consumers are cautioned about possible serious or life-threatening side effects, associated with certain antidepressants, particularly an increased risk for suicide.

Mental illnesses are complicated, and finding the most effective medication is a complex process. Please bear in mind that this process is often one of trial and error, depending on individual responses to medications. It would be helpful to both you and your young adult to anticipate questions that might be posed during the first appointment with a psychiatric provider. Your adult child will be asked for a description of their current symptoms as well as past symptoms, if applicable. If your young adult has received prior treatment, the current provider will want to know the name of the medication(s), the length of time the medication was taken and the dose, any side effects as well as benefits from the medication, and the reason the medication was discontinued. Additionally, a list of medications your adult child is currently taking is important to provide. If you or other family members have been tried on or currently take medication for a similar disorder, this information could be immensely beneficial to your adult child's treatment. However, our experience as clinicians has taught us that many emerging adults and older adults do not keep records of previous medications.

Psychotropic medications increase your adult child's ability to manage the symptoms associated with serious anxiety, depression, and bipolar disorder. Treatment often entails the use of various combinations of medications at different stages of the illness. For example, the psychopharmacological treatment of bipolar I disorder involves four main categories of medications that may be used in various combinations: mood stabilizers, antipsychotics, antianxiety medications, and antidepressants. Again, the prescriber must have a high level of expertise to determine which medications to use and how to combine these. They must also be mindful of side effects and interactions with additional medications your emerging adult may be taking for other medical and psychological conditions. For a list of medications used to treat anxiety, depression, and bipolar disorder, see Table 6.3.

TABLE 6.3. Medications Used to Treat Mental Illnesses

Disorder	Type of medication	Examples
Generalized anxiety disorder	Selective serotonin reuptake inhibitors (SSRIs): antidepressants	Celexa (citalopram) Lexapro (escitalopram) Paxil (paroxetine) Zoloft (sertraline)
	Serotonin-epinephrine reuptake inhibitors (SNRIs): antidepressants	Effexor (venlafazine) Pristiq (desvenlafaxine) Cymbalta (duloxetine)
	Benzodiazepines (used primarily to treat acute anxiety/panic attacks)	Xanax (alprazolam) Ativan (lorazepam) Valium (diazepam)
	Beta-blockers (used to treat performance anxiety)	Inderal (propranolol)
Major depressive disorder	Selective serotonin reuptake inhibitors (SSRIs): antidepressants	Celexa (citalopram) Lexapro (escitalopram) Prozac (fluoxetine) Vibryd (vilazodone) Zoloft (sertraline)
	Serotonin-epinephrine reuptake inhibitors (SNRIs): antidepressants	Effexor (venlafaxine) Pristiq (desvenlafaxine) Cymbalta (duloxetine)
	Atypical antidepressants	Trintellix (vortioxetine) Wellbutrin (bupropion) Remeron (mirtazapine)
	Tricyclic (TCAs), first-generation antidepressants	Elavil (amitriptyline) Tofranil (imipramine) Pamelor (nortriptyline)

TABLE 6.3. **Medications Used to Treat Mental Illnesses** *(Continued)*

Disorder	Type of medication	Examples
	Monoamine oxidase inhibitors (MAOIs)	Marplan (isocarboxazid) Nardil (phenelzine) Parnate (tranylcypromine)
Bipolar disorder	Mood stabilizers	Lithium Depakote (divalproex sodium) Lamictal (lamotrigine) Tegretol (carbamazepine)
	Antipsychotics	Zyprexa (olanzapine) Abilify (aripiprazole) Seroquel (quetiapine) Geodon (ziprasidone) Risperdal (risperidone) Saphris (asenapine) Latuda (lurasidone) Vraylar (cariprazine)
Mania/hypomania	Lithium and Seroquel (quetiapine) tops the list for all three phases of the illness: mania, depression, and the maintenance phase	
Mania, with psychosis	Lithium	
Depression	Lithium Latuda (Lurasidone) Lamictal (Lamotrigine) Seroquel (quetiapine)	

OTHER FORMS OF TREATMENT

Two popular treatment options for young adults experiencing depression, anxiety, and other forms of psychological distress are exercise and the use of creative arts. Both are backed by research for their effectiveness, especially as an addition to the talk therapy approaches presented in this chapter.

Exercise is an appealing option for emerging adults for several reasons. Strong evidence now establishes that regular moderate-to-vigorous aerobic (vigorous walking, swimming, biking, etc.) and anaerobic (sprinting, weightlifting, etc.) exercise for a minimum of 30 minutes 5 days a week produces antidepressant and antianxiety effects in young adults (Singh et al., 2023). It could prove especially beneficial given the tendency toward the intake of high fat, salt, and sweets and the more sedentary lifestyles often observed in this age group. Exercise is also especially appealing for young adults because it holds the possibility of improving body image and gaining control over one's body in a healthy way. From a brain health perspective, engaging in regular moderate-level exercise increases levels of natural mood-enhancing brain chemicals (e.g., serotonin, dopamine, and other neurotransmitters; endorphins) and supports healthy cell development in the brain (de Sousa Fernandes et al., 2020).

You may have heard about something called BDNF (brain-derived neurotrophic factor) in connection with exercise. Simply stated, this is a brain chemical which exercise has been shown to increase, and which has a positive effect on mood (Murawska-Ciałowicz et al., 2021). When we couple this with the positive effects of exercise on overall health, it strengthens our suggestion that physical activity is an important component in the treatment options for young adults.

Creative arts and expressive therapies have long been used with children and are now being more commonly used with adults. These include art therapy, music therapy, drama therapy, dance movement therapy, poetry therapy, and expressive arts therapies which typically use a combination of different art forms. Creative activities help emerging adults develop a greater capacity to self-reflect and to gain personal insight. They also increase the young adult's ability to focus their attention and to manage stress, anxiety, and depression more effectively (Smriti et al., 2022). Lastly, these creative therapies enhance the adult child's coping skills relative to emotional trauma (Baker et al., 2018).

Despite public interest and widespread media attention on the use of psychedelics (e.g., psilocybin ["magic mushrooms"], LSD [lysergic acid diethylamide], peyote, ayahuasca, and DMT [dimethyltryptamine]) to treat depression, anxiety, posttraumatic distress, and substance abuse, the American Psychiatric Association has not endorsed their use, citing a need for more research support (Alpert et al., 2022). Currently, the National Institute on Drug Abuse is conducting research on these substances to gain a better understanding of the health effects of psychedelic and dissociative drugs, how they work in the brain, and whether they may be able to treat substance use disorders and other conditions. Esketamine (a.k.a., ketamine), a dissociative psychedelic drug, was approved by the FDA in 2019 for use in treatment-resistant depression; it is the only FDA-approved psychedelic treatment.

HOW TO SUPPORT YOUR ADULT CHILD WHILE THEY CONSIDER OR BEGIN TREATMENT

In this section, we focus on the skills that are necessary for your role as an advanced coach as your young adult both considers and agrees to begin treatment (see Exhibit 6.1). When your young adult has a serious mental health issue, one of the most important skills you can have is educating yourself about treatment options. We have

> **EXHIBIT 6.1.** Additional Advanced Coaching Skills for When Your Adult Child Has a Mental Health Issue
>
> • Educate yourself about treatment options.
> • Educate yourself about ambivalence.
> • Practice the "spirit of motivational interviewing."
> • Consider using a patient advocate.
> • Understand HIPAA.
> • Be prepared for crisis situations.
> • Monitor your own mental health.
>
> *Note.* HIPAA = Health Insurance Portability and Accountability Act.

already provided information to get you started with this skill. But how helpful will this information be if your emerging adult refuses to get help? This leads us to a second critical skill: educating yourself about your young adult's ambivalence. The process of finding help can be very frustrating for you as a parent and result in a power struggle with your adult child. We will give you tools to help you communicate with your young adult about their ambivalence to seek and stay in treatment.

Educate Yourself About Your Young Adult's Ambivalence

We turn our attention now to helping you as a parent understand the range of reactions your young adult may have to the prospect of seeking treatment. Based on our research and clinical experience, we estimate that approximately one-third of emerging adults with symptoms of anxiety, depression, bipolarity, and other disorders are agreeable to the prospect of engaging in treatment and are open to their parents' assistance in finding appropriate mental health services. Roughly one-third of emerging adults are ambivalent about seeking treatment. This means their willingness to participate in treatment may fluctuate from time to time. They might experience interest in having parents assist them with the process of finding appropriate treatment resources. The remaining third may be firmly resistant to the idea of treatment. When young adults are ambivalent or refuse to get treatment all together, it can feel like being on an emotional roller coaster for many parents. Parents often mistake their adult child's ambivalence for resistance; the latter connotes opposition to treatment, and the former refers to the simultaneous desire and reluctance to engage in treatment. Most therapists view ambivalence and resistance as natural and universal and believe that neither are problematic, especially when viewed from the lens of the young adults' readiness for change (Miller & Rollnick, 2002). Let's take a look at a model of change that may help you further understand your young adult's reluctance and waffling behaviors around entering and sticking with treatment.

STAGES OF CHANGE

Considering how hard it can be for any of us to make a change in our behavior, perhaps the Stages of Change model (Prochaska & DiClemente, 1983) could be of use here. This model originally described how people approach a major behavioral change, such as ending alcohol misuse. The model includes five stages: precontemplation, contemplation, preparation, action, and maintenance. See Exhibit 6.2 for a description of these stages.

Imagine you want to make a change, such as starting a diet, engaging in a regular exercise program, or eliminating caffeine from your diet; you move through these stages, but not necessarily in a linear fashion. Clearly, until you recognize that there is an issue requiring your attention, there will be no movement. The stages can occur in cycles, and you can be stuck in a stage or revisit a stage

---

> **EXHIBIT 6.2.** Stages of Change Model
>
> • Precontemplation: "The problem is not on my radar."
> • Contemplation: "I guess there's a problem, but I'm not ready to do anything."
> • Preparation: "I have a problem, and I'm getting ready to do something about it."
> • Action: "I'm taking steps to deal with my problem."
> • Maintenance: "I want to hold onto the changes and keep the momentum going."

---

multiple times before moving on to the next one. And for some of us, we may not progress past the precontemplation stage because ambivalence about wanting to change stalls us in our tracks.

The Stages of Change model helps us to appreciate the role that ambivalence plays in any behavioral change, and, when combined with what we know about the weak executive function skills in many young adults, it's no wonder that your adult child may be reluctant at best to move off of square one and take action. For example, in Chapter 4, we read about Anne's journey starting from her outright refusal to acknowledge a problem to her eventual willingness to follow through with a consultation with her general practitioner.

REASONS FOR AMBIVALENCE

There are many reasons for your adult child's reluctance to engage in treatment, including their lack of practical experience making health care decisions. When your adult child turns 18 years old, they need to transition from the pediatric to the adult system. Many young adults simultaneously choose to shift away from relying on their parents to make their decisions and are now in charge of their own health care. When your adult child develops symptoms of a mental illness, they are expected to make important and complex decisions about mental health treatment on their own.

Another reason for resisting getting help is simply that they don't believe there is anything wrong. Given the lack of mature reasoning skills and their desire to fit in with their peers, they may often ignore the symptoms and continue with life as usual. They might also resist the pressure of a parent to suggest, cajole, or insist that they see someone. Just as you may instinctively move into caretaker mode to try and arrange things for them, so do they often push back asserting their adult status and cutting you off from lending a hand. As we discussed in Chapter 3, many young adults are in denial about their symptoms and cope through substance misuse or other impulsive and risky behaviors. The prospect of talk therapy or medication for these young adults is fraught with ambivalence; they realize something is wrong, but they are not yet ready to consider formal mental health treatment.

Young adults may also fear change and have concerns about being judged. They worry about the impact of being in treatment on their relationships with friends. Emerging adults often fear being perceived by their peers as incapable or inadequate. These qualities are the antithesis of how they want to be seen and how they want to see themselves.

In addition to the developmental need of this age group to feel and to be seen as capable and adequate, young adults who are people of color and/or LGBTQ have additional reasons for being distrustful of mental health institutions and services. Marginalization and discrimination have contributed to problems with the lack of affordability and access to evidence-based mental health care services and reinforce the ambivalence that young adults of color and/or LGBTQ young adults continue to experience about treatment.

Stigma is another reason a young adult may be spooked by the idea of treatment. Even though mental health issues are much more publicly acknowledged and discussed these days, the stigma looms large in the minds of many. Young adults are not immune to this kind of thinking. To make matters worse, if one or both parents work in a helping profession or have friends who do, the young adult may feel their privacy could be violated if they sought help in their community. Many young adults are apprehensive about the possible impact of a mental health diagnosis on their career or academic record. This is a concern that parents, including you, might also share.

Parents Can Be Ambivalent, Too!

We also have to recognize that parents, like emerging adults, often have their own mixed feelings about therapy. As a parent, you may be skeptical about the effectiveness of therapy and believe that emotional issues are best handled within the family. Seeking mental health treatment may even be considered a weakness. For parents who are people of color and/or LGBT, the history of discrimination and mistreatment by the medical community can get in the way of seeking and valuing mental health services. In any case, it may be your own misgivings about therapy that influence your adult child's decision regarding seeking treatment.

If in the past you had reason to seek mental health services for your child or adolescent, that experience will likely color the current situation for better and for worse. You might have been less than satisfied with your experience; perhaps the office staff or even the providers were not particularly helpful and responsive and may have even insinuated that your parenting style was not up to snuff. These are certainly reasons to be less than enthusiastic about the process of seeking treatment now. On the other hand, if your experience with mental health services was positive, you may be more inclined to return. Regardless of where you are on the continuum, equipping yourself with knowledge and strategies to navigate the complexities of today's mental health system will pay off.

WHEN AMBIVALENCE COMES AND GOES

Even if your emerging adult decides to begin treatment, this doesn't mean they will stick with it. Your adult child must feel a connection with their therapist for therapy to be effective. Most clients develop a sense of the unspoken chemistry that exists with their particular therapist during the first or second session. Young adults may prefer their therapist to be of a particular gender, age, ethnicity, and sexual orientation, for example. Research has shown that the quality of the therapeutic relationship is a key determinant in the success of treatment (Flückiger et al., 2018; Norcross & Lambert, 2018). If your young adult expresses ambivalence or dissatisfaction or if you sense uncertainty, you might encourage them to consider someone else.

At the same time, it's important to understand that therapy is a process. It is important to bear in mind that effective treatment for your adult child may involve different levels of treatment. The provider must be well trained, skilled, and ethical, and perhaps most importantly, they must also be the right fit for your young adult and their needs. Even when a connection with the therapist is solid, there will be times when your young adult may feel angry or upset with their therapist. What your young adult needs to do is process these feelings with their therapist and to grow through their conversation. Therapy has the potential to be most effective if these ups and downs can be anticipated. We want to be very clear that with the right fit between therapist and client, therapy can and does work.

Just as young adults may be ambivalent about entering and staying in treatment, they may also be ambivalent about taking or continuing medication(s). It is common for adults who are diagnosed with mental disorders, especially bipolar disorder, to stop taking their medications at some point against medical advice (Semahegn et al., 2020). This would include emerging adults. In many instances, when they start to feel better, their lack of insight gets in the way of their ability to realize that their medications are helping. Unfortunately, the practice of discontinuing their medication puts young adults at high risk for recurrence of bipolar symptoms and for slower recovery. Each time an emerging adult relapses, they are more vulnerable to future and more severe mood episodes.

In some cases, emerging adults become impatient and discouraged when results are not immediate; antidepressants can take as long as 2 to 6 weeks to become effective. As you have already learned, patience is not a strong suit for many young adults. The failure to take medications as prescribed, is termed *nonadherence*. Adherence, particularly among emerging adults, can fluctuate over time for various reasons, including practical ones like forgetting to take medication, costs, and confusion about instructions, for example. Young adults may also experience noxious side effects associated with their medications, including weight gain, jitteriness, and acne, among others, which can contribute to nonadherence. Other issues that impact adherence include psychological factors (e.g., disbelief of having a mental illness) and co-occurring substance misuse or attention-deficit/hyperactivity disorder, for example.

Let's hear some more about Jessie's ambivalence to get help, as told by Jessie's mom, Rachel.

> Jessie's anxiety was getting worse. I could tell by the frequent phone calls and pressured tone I heard in her voice. Plus, I now know that she missed three days of work. Whenever I suggested that she get some help, she would laugh it off.
>
> "Work is crazy right now, Mom. You know how it gets when five different people want you to do something, and all at

the same time. It's nothing new, and I can handle it. Really. I'm just calling to check in and see how you and Jared are doing."

I reminded her of the breathing exercises we had practiced together in the past when she was feeling stressed and asked if she wanted me to come over and do them with her. She laughed it off and said "No thanks! I'm not that bad off!"

Nevertheless, the calls kept coming until finally one day, I'd heard enough. Jessie called to say she was taking a few days off from work.

"I've been feeling really tired lately, and I haven't been sleeping well. My boss says he can cover for me. I just need some rest. It's, well . . . you know, a good idea I guess."

She sounded less wound up, but also very lethargic to me. In my work with the EMT squad, I'd seen my fair share of mental health issues, and I knew Jessie struggled with anxiety a lot—and likely also with depression at times, although that was not as prominent in her symptoms.

"Jessie, I really think it would be helpful if you talked with someone about what you are going through. There are some good folks in town who work with young adults, and . . ."

Before I could finish, she was in defense mode.

"Come on, mom. I already told you I don't need to 'talk to' anyone. I am not some crazy nut ball that you have to haul to the hospital. I won't see anyone in town because they all know you. I couldn't trust them to keep anything a secret. They probably talk with each other about the psychos they work with. And they already know me, most of them. No way."

Jessie was practically in tears at this point, which only raised my stress level further. She was not one to cry or get emotional very often. Her outburst was disconcerting, and I was concerned that things were escalating. I tried to calm her down, suggesting that we talk again the next morning to see how she was doing.

"Maybe, but no more of this treatment crap, okay?"

I knew I couldn't promise that, so instead I suggested she get some rest, and I'd talk with her in the morning.

I hung up the phone with a heavy feeling in my gut.

Rachel is clearly worried about her daughter. She has some knowledge of the mental health issues Jessie is struggling with, and she knows the importance of getting some help. However, she is also keenly aware that Jessie is an adult, and therefore, she cannot be led into treatment unwillingly unless she poses a danger to herself or to others.

It appears that Jessie is waffling between the precontemplation and the contemplation stage; although she is aware of her symptoms at times, she is in denial of her symptoms at other times. The ambivalence she feels is a normal part of the process. It also helps to explain the back-and-forth between stages as well as the time it can take to reach the final stage. In addition to gaining an understanding of where Jessie is in the stages of change, it may also benefit Rachel to learn how to communicate with her daughter in a way that doesn't create a power struggle or standoff.

As a parent, you don't need specialized training to know your adult child is in trouble. Your gut feeling may serve you well. Rachel's concern for Jessie is apparent, as is her desire to help her daughter. She is torn between staying out of Jessie's way and moving in to convince her to do something. It's hard to know whether to butt in to your young adult's life or to maintain a wait-and-see approach. If your young adult lives away from home and at some distance, it may complicate matters further because you likely have limited information on how things are going for them. Fortunately for Rachel, she and Jessie are in the same small community, so she has more access to what might be happening. She doesn't have the full picture, though, as we shall soon see.

> Rather than call Jessie the next morning and forgetting that she said she was taking a few days off, I decided to surprise her at her workplace around lunchtime and take her out for a bite to eat. I knew her schedule allowed for a lunch break, and I figured she would be less inclined to get angry at me in her

workplace. I drove to the Planet Fitness location and walked in just before noon. Her boss was there and gave me a confused smile as I approached the desk.

"Hi Jordan," I said to him. "I came to surprise Jessie and take her to lunch."

He looked around uncomfortably, before motioning me to the alcove behind the front desk. "Uh, Rachel," he began. "I, uh . . . had to let Jessie go last week. Well, temporarily at least. She was missing work, and not able to concentrate when she was here. We're into the fall rush, and she couldn't keep up with what she needed to do. I really like her, and I hope she can come back at some point. But it just wasn't working. I'm sorry, I thought she would've told you." He looked embarrassed, but not more so than I felt. My cheeks burned as I took in what he was telling me. Jessie was fired last week, and I knew nothing about it.

"I . . . it's okay Jordan. She doesn't live at home, so I don't see her every day. She probably just hasn't had time to let me know." I lied, knowing full well that my daughter had made a deliberate decision to shut me out of what had happened.

"I really am sorry, Rachel. Please tell her I hope she can get herself together and come back soon."

"Thanks, Jordan. I have to go, errands to run, you know." I turned quickly and headed back out the door. I was pissed off, worried, and embarrassed. Most of all I was hurt that my daughter didn't come to me and let me know what had happened. How was I going to approach her knowing that her situation was even worse than I had thought? And how was I going to convince my daughter to get the help she clearly needed? Her situation was getting worse, and I felt helpless. My stress meter was ready to explode as I drove out of the parking lot and headed home. In addition to everything else about the situation, I was concerned that Jessie would not be able to afford her apartment without a job and wondered how I would be able to support her on top of providing for Jared. Money was always tight, but I managed to keep a healthy savings account for emergencies. This could potentially drain my reserves.

Rachel is clearly angry and at her wit's end. She worries about Jessie's refusal to get some help and can't understand why. Perhaps it would be helpful if Rachel took a different perspective on her daughter's situation.

Practice the "Spirit of Motivational Interviewing"

Motivational interviewing is an approach first developed by Miller and Rollnick (2002) in their work with people struggling with addictions. It has since been applied to a wide range of issues as a way of fostering communication. For our purposes, motivational interviewing is, at its heart, a "motivation conversation" between parent and adult child, with the aim of supporting your adult child's personal commitment to change. It involves the following elements: compassion, collaboration, autonomy support, and drawing on the young adult's inner resources needed for change. We find that these attributes are consistent with our definition of an advanced coach.

This approach builds on many of the skills that are already in your tote bag (e.g., listen intently; use clear, deliberate communication). Additional skills specific to motivational interviewing are open-ended questions and statements, affirmations, reflections, and summaries (see Table 6.4).

Let's return to Rachel's situation with Jessie and her refusal to seek treatment because mom knew "all the professionals in town." After learning of her daughter's job loss, Rachel moves from a wait-and-see posture to a more proactive stance, however, she recognizes that Jessie needs autonomy support. Equipped with an understanding of stages of change and with the communication skills needed to address her daughter's ambivalence, Rachel engages in a dialogue with Jessie. In this discussion, Rachel uses the skills associated with the "spirit of motivational interviewing." She listens to Jessie's story, despite her own fears and concerns about her daughter. Rachel

TABLE 6.4. "Spirit of Motivational Interviewing" Skills

Skill	Purpose	Examples
Open-ended questions and statements	Explore topics in an unstructured and in-depth way	"How would you like things to be different?" "When you think about treatment, what stops you from considering it?" "Tell me more about what you feel on your 'down' days."
Affirmations	Demonstrate appreciation and understanding of the other person's strengths	"If I were in your shoes, I don't know if I could have managed nearly so well." "You've overcome obstacles before and I admire you for that." "You participated in counseling when you were younger and you quickly learned how to adjust to change."
Reflections	Demonstrate that you are interested in, and listening to, what the other person is saying	"It appears that . . ." "It sounds like you . . ." "What you seem to be saying is . . ." "Correct me if I'm wrong, but it seems to me . . ."
Summaries	Gather more information, pull it together in a coherent way, and show that you are listening and that you care	"Here is what I've heard . . ." "Tell me if I've missed anything . . ." "Let's see if I can summarize what you just said."

responds with empathy and support, which enables Jessie to confide in her mom. Note that Rachel ends this dialogue with an invitation to follow-up. She asks Jessie to contemplate possible options and offers her help if Jessie needs it. Consistent with her role as advanced coach, Rachel attempts to support Jessie's autonomy as much as possible, even in the presence of a possible anxiety or mood disorder. Rachel also sees her own behavior in a new light. Jessie pointed out that she wasn't available, and that hurt; it also gave her the opportunity to examine her own behavior and make a course correction (see story below).

Let's see how this might play out as Rachel pulls up outside Jessie's apartment after spending a couple hours walking by the lake near their town. She has calmed her breathing and shaken off much of the anger she felt leaving Jessie's workplace.

I walked up to the door of Jessie's apartment, took a deep breath and knocked. I heard footsteps moving toward the door, and then Jessie appeared through the space between the chain and the door frame.

"Hi, Jess. May I come in?"

Jessie eyed me suspiciously for a moment, then slid the chair back and stepped aside. I entered the kitchen and took in the disarray and empty food containers. She moved to the table and sat down. Ignoring the mess, I sat opposite her. "How are you doing?"

She shrugged her shoulders.

"I went to the Planet Fitness to see if you wanted to go out to lunch," I began . . .

"Oh crap, so Jordan told you." She moaned. "He had no right . . ."

I held up my hand to silence her. "He's worried about you, Jess, and so am I. I'm here . . . talk to me." I sat back and waited.

She looked at me for a minute, then down at the floor. "Yeah, well, you aren't here very much. You're always off on emergency runs. I'm sorry I didn't tell you about being fired.

I just thought it was a bad dream and anyway you wouldn't be around to talk to. I've tried to get another job, but so far, no luck. I can't concentrate on anything, and I feel so anxious all the time. I feel like I'm losing my mind, Mom. What's wrong with me?"

"Jessie, I don't know, but I do see how upset and scared you are right now, and it sounds like you're mad at me for not being available earlier when you needed to talk [empathy]. I know you don't want to see anyone in town but . . ."

Being human, and a mom who doesn't know what else to do, I started to offer the suggestion of seeing a therapist again. Of course it bombed.

"Don't start that crap again. I am NOT seeing someone in town! I already told you!"

"Okay, I hear you. Sounds like things are getting worse lately, though. I'd like to hear more about what happened at work?"

"Jordan was really sorry, but he said that I missed too many days of work." She trails off with tears in her eyes.

"You know, Jess, I think it takes a strong person to have felt the way you have and still keep on going to work for so long [affirmation]. I also know that it's up to you to decide what you want to do next."

Jessie shook her head. "I feel stuck, Mom. I don't know what to do. But I don't want to stay stuck. What should I do?"

"You've always been a go-getter Jess, and yet you just lost your job. How does that fit with your goal of being a manager and maybe future business owner? Being stuck isn't fun! I felt that way after your dad died. I couldn't imagine how to move on. Talking with someone who could be objective really helped me. It might be helpful for you, too."

"Okay, Mom, I get what you're saying. I'll see someone, but just not here in town."

"I have an idea, Jess. There are service providers online who can help you. They aren't in this town, or even close by, some of them. And they will not know me or anyone here. So you can be sure the whole town is not going to know your business."

"Internet shrinks? Never heard of that." She chewed on her lower lip for a moment. "Let me think about it, okay?"

"It's your decision, Jess. Let me know if I can help."

I stood up and prepared to leave. Jessie got up and gave me a big hug. "I thought you were going to yell at me. Thanks for not doing that."

I walked out the door, a small smile forming on my lips. The situation was far from settled, but this felt like a baby step in the right direction. I have to admit, I was feeling a bit inside-out myself at this point. Hoping that Jessie would agree to try telehealth, wishing that none of this was real. But it was. I was also kicking myself for not being as available as I thought I was.

As Rachel showed us in the dialogue, it is the natural tendency for a parent to want to make things "right" by directing their adult child and telling them what they "need" and/or what they "should" do. This is known as the "righting reflex," and something likely familiar to most parents (Miller & Rollnick, 2012). However, the more parents direct and tell their adult child to get help, the more they might dig in their heels.

Finding a telehealth provider who works with young adults might be the solution for Jessie and others who are refusing to seek help due to privacy concerns. Rachel opened her tote bag and pulled out some of the skills we put in there (e.g., empathic listening, non-judgmental interaction, and autonomy support). Rachel also was able to center herself and remained calm while she talked with her daughter.

Consider Using a Patient Advocate

Jessie seems to be in fairly good communication with her mom, Rachel, and has at least agreed to think about getting some help. The story of Anne and Claire is quite different. In Chapters 4 and 5, Claire described Anne's ambivalence about treatment. Although

Claire knew that Anne was getting some form of psychotropic medication, she was left in the dark about who her provider was and what sort of medication she was taking. Anne decided on her own to try various medications over the course of 8 to 10 months. Claire's feelings of powerlessness were palpable as she watched Anne's symptoms worsen. Finally, Anne was involuntarily hospitalized during a manic episode, and she was diagnosed with bipolar I disorder.

Claire's story illustrates the potential value of having a responsible adult aiding the process of finding appropriate treatment. It stands to reason that these decisions are difficult; navigating the mental health care system and finding appropriate treatment is a challenge in the best of circumstances. Young adults generally lack the specialized skills and often the resources they might need to find quality treatment. When the symptoms of serious mental health issues are added to the mix, the insight and skill set of the young adult are even more compromised.

Given that Anne does not want her parents involved in her treatment, there are potential benefits of inviting another person to serve as her advocate. This could be a different family member or other mature adult. We stress that the advocate is someone whom the young adult trusts. This is different from a health surrogate, which is a legally binding relationship. Claire would gladly step aside and let this advocate guide her daughter through the process of finding treatment. As a parent, she is willing to trust this person to serve as a primary support for Anne. It is vitally important that the advocate has a certain skill set, which ironically is the same skill set as the advanced coach.

An adult who assumes the role of advocate must have previously gained the trust of your adult child; they must be accessible and available and have the capacity to remain calm yet be able to communicate assertively. It is also helpful for your young adult's advocate to be familiar with mental health services and how to navigate the system. It is important that clear boundaries be established at the start of this relationship. For example, it is imperative that the advocate not make decisions for your emerging adult or be judgmental about decisions they make. An advocate must be able to listen, find additional information and resources, and possibly transport your adult child to appointments. As treatment progresses, the advocate also checks in with your young adult periodically to observe any ill effects (e.g., side effects of medications, their reactions to the counseling process). Any information about the nature of the treatment, including medication, that is disclosed to the advocate, does not get passed along to you without your young adult's permission.

The relationship with an advocate, then, requires that ground rules be firmly established at the beginning. All parties should understand and respect the boundaries. This means that information about the young adult's mental health care is confidential and not disclosed without the expressed permission of that young adult. The use of a patient health care advocate is a well-established practice in the medical field. We acknowledge that it may be challenging for parents to see someone else in this role. However, we believe the complex and fragmented nature of mental health care services today demands that when a loved one needs treatment, they need an advocate.

Be Prepared for Crisis Situations

This is easy to say and often difficult to do. How do you as a parent prepare for a crisis? First, a mental health crisis is any situation in which a person experiences severe psychological distress coupled with a crippling inability to function. This puts them at risk of harming themselves or others. As a parent, it is vital that you realize this is possible and often likely to occur with a serious mental illness.

It is important to support the autonomy of young adults with serious mental health issues, especially in times of crisis. One way to do this is by completing a crisis plan and/or a psychiatric advance directive (PAD). Crisis plans are written plans that are developed to identify and resolve any future crisis that might arise. These plans are prepared with the active involvement of your adult child during a period of stability. They should include early warning signs that your adult child may be heading into a mental health crisis as well as coping strategies that can be used. If your young adult is incapable of implementing the coping strategies, you may want to request the assistance of the advocate. Additional information should include your adult child's demographic and diagnostic information, the names and contact information for persons identified by your adult child as part of their support network, as well as medications, and treatment choices. More information can be found online (https://mhanational.org/crisis-planning-caregivers).

PADs are legally binding and include specific documents that detail your emerging adult's preferences for forms of treatment, types of medications, specific in-patient facilities, and other concerns in the event that they are unable to make decisions or speak for themselves when they are in a manic, psychotic, or confused mental state (Substance Abuse and Mental Health Services Administration, 2019). An excellent resource for parents and their emerging adults regarding state-by-state requirements and downloadable forms for PADs can be found online (https://mhanational.org/creating-psychiatric-advance-directive). Not only do crisis plans and PADs help protect young adults from unwanted treatment, they also help promote dialogue between family members about the young adult's diagnosis, treatment experiences, and personal needs.

Monitor Your Own Mental Health

As the parent of a young adult in severe psychological distress, you pivot back and forth among the roles of caretaker, coach, and advanced coach. This process can be mentally, physically, and emotionally exhausting. More than any other time in your parenting journey, you need to make yourself a priority. This involves monitoring all aspects of your overall well-being, particularly your own mental health. Being there for your emerging adult is demanding and time-consuming, and you need to be in a good place regardless of your role. We encourage you to continue practicing the breathing and grounding exercises and to use the tools in your tote bag.

As therapists, we strongly recommend that you consider finding a therapist for yourself and maybe encourage your partner, if applicable, to do the same. We have talked at some length in this chapter about the benefits for your young adult of seeking treatment. We believe that having an objective person to help you sort through your own feelings and challenges in this situation can be extremely valuable. Similar to your young adult, finding a compatible mental health provider to help you navigate your experience is an important tool to keep in mind. We will continue to provide information specific to maintaining and improving your mental health. One step in the process may simply be getting some therapy yourself.

SUMMARY

Your young adult's job of finding effective mental health treatment in a post-COVID world is rendered more formidable than ever due to shortages of mental health providers, underfunding of mental health services, and other factors. Besides obvious considerations such as affordability, geographic proximity, scheduling needs and availability, and therapists' credentials and expertise, it is essential that your adult child's provider(s) be the right fit for them. However, your young adult may have neither the motivation nor the skills necessary to make wise decisions about mental health care providers and treatment options. If you, as a parent, are unable to assist in this process, you might want to discuss with your emerging adult the option of asking another family member or trusted friend to serve in an advocacy role. Because the treatment of anxiety, depression, bipolar, and other related disorders demands such a high level of expertise and experience, the decision about mental health practitioners requires thoughtful and informed consideration. Additionally, emerging adults and parents should be aware of the complex nature of psychopharmacological treatment. It is essential that your young adult and you, or their mental health advocate, work actively to monitor side effects and unwanted changes accompanying the use of medications.

We hope that if your adult child needs professional help, they get it. And we hope that the help is actually helpful—that it effectively relieves symptoms—thereby decreasing distress and improving functioning. If or when this happens, consider pivoting to the next role: wise counsel. We will discuss this new role in the next chapter.

POINTS TO POCKET

- Beware: Accurate diagnosis and effective treatment can truly make a critical difference in your adult child's future. Your ability to choose providers wisely is vital.
- Please remember: "Asking for help is never a sign of weakness. It's one of the bravest things you can do. And it can save your life" (Collins, 2017, p. 127).
- The fit between your young adult and their therapist is the best predictor of success in therapy.
- Stand up for your young adult. Our mental health care system demands that we be a strong voice for ourselves and our emerging adults in psychological distress, who may not be equipped to act as their own advocate.
- A caveat: The most highly recommended treatment mode is talk therapy plus medication (when needed).

CHAPTER 7

BECOMING WISE COUNSEL

In any given moment we have two options: To step forward into growth or to step back into safety.

—Abraham Maslow

We recognize that in the last few chapters, we have focused on more serious mental health issues and even crisis situations. It is important to understand that while many emerging adults do experience high levels of psychological distress or diagnosed conditions, there is a sizable number who don't. We believe what is most important to a parent in determining how they respond is their young adult's level of stability and functioning.

In this chapter, we focus on situations in which young adults' experience of psychological distress is of lesser intensity (e.g., mild-to-moderate distress) and their functioning appears to be in the moderate range. As we arrive on the brink of another pivot, we think it would be helpful to reinforce the concept of the parent pivoting wheel and remind you that these shifts don't happen in a linear fashion. You pivot to meet the needs of your young adult in their current situation.

RETURNING TO THE MENTAL HEALTH ISSUE CONTINUUM

Keep in mind that mental health issues fall along a continuum, and psychological distress is present to varying degrees in all emerging adults. Returning to our stories of young adults and their families, we find Anne diagnosed with bipolar illness and experiencing an acute phase of her illness that lands her in the hospital. This is clearly a mental health crisis for her and vicariously for her parents. However, remember that with the correct diagnosis and effective treatment, she is capable of reaching a period of stability in which she can successfully sustain and nurture friendships as well as family relationships and recommit to her studies. Claire and Stan could then approach Anne from a very different perspective, one that continues to support her journey toward greater autonomy. We acknowledge that bipolar illness can be extremely challenging with periods of depression and mania often recurring. The necessity of being prepared for this possibility is important for Claire and Stan. It is vital to keep the parent pivoting wheel greased to adapt as Anne's situation changes. We know this is not easy. Stan and Claire may want to stay in caretaker mode, afraid to let their guard down in case of a recurrence. This is an understandable response. However, in the long run, engaging in autonomy support behaviors will be more beneficial for all concerned.

In contrast, Ian's story is an example of a young adult who exhibits mild-to-moderate levels of psychological distress. His use of the internet became problematic as a coping tool when his anxiety and apprehension about the future intensified. Pete's natural inclination was to jump in as caretaker, and he even went so far as to threaten to take away all of Ian's screens. Although Ian's behaviors were alarming to Pete as his dad, objectively speaking, they didn't rise to the level of Anne's symptoms and behaviors. Therefore, you might anticipate Pete having less of a need to pivot to a caretaker role, or for that matter to stay in the advanced coach role. In this chapter, you will learn how Pete assumes a very different parenting role on the pivoting wheel, one that supports Ian's growing need for autonomy.

Regardless of where a young adult is on the continuum of mental health issues, a universal tool for parents is education. From the beginning of the book, we have been educating you regarding the emerging adult culture, mental health issues, and treatment options. The more knowledge you have, the more empowered and confident you will feel to assist your young adult and to cope effectively with whatever the situation may present. Remember, psychological distress is a part of the emerging adult experience regardless of whether they have a diagnosable mental illness. Understanding this allows you to be less reactive to every little thing. You will have a clearer sense of when trouble may be brewing, requiring you to pivot to a different role.

PIVOTING TO WISE COUNSEL

The wise counsel role builds on the skills that are already a part of your tote bag. In the role of advanced coach, you equipped yourself with the information necessary to guide your emerging adult through the challenging process of finding effective mental health treatment. Your young adult, however, will make the decisions they believe will best meet their needs. They may or may not opt to seek and remain in therapy. They may or not agree to take medication. They may or may not be ambivalent for some time about the decision to seek treatment. Regardless of which scenario you are facing with your emerging adult, you have learned to communicate with them in ways that encourage and support them as they navigate this unfamiliar and intimidating territory. Change can be uncomfortable and scary for all involved. You have the skills to support their autonomy, but you remain ready and able to pivot to a caretaker role should your young adult verbalize or behave in ways that signal a possible mental health crisis.

As a wise counsel, you will act as an on-call consultant for your young adult. Each of the previous skills you have learned in this book are prerequisites for entering this role. You will now be emotionally available whenever they ask for your input. A wise counsel is also equipped to communicate effectively, particularly in difficult and challenging circumstances. As you will learn in this chapter, parents in the wise counsel role are able to look at their young adult's situations and relationships through a systemic lens. That is, they see the big picture and are more likely to appreciate the complex and interrelated nature of relationships. When in wise counsel mode, the parent is able to recognize that at times their adult child's symptoms and behaviors may be triggering for them as parents, and they are able to step back from responding. They are rather better equipped to confront emotional injuries from the past that can be triggered when they interact with their adult children. The skills we present in this chapter are all incrementally more complex and more challenging to understand and use than those we presented in previous chapters. They require considerable time and practice.

Let's turn now to the additional skills for your tote bag that will be necessary as you pivot from advanced coach to wise counsel. As you see listed in Exhibit 7.1, there are several tools to help you navigate the road ahead in your role as wise counsel.

EXHIBIT 7.1. How to Be a Wise Counsel for Your Adult Child
• Practice radical acceptance. • Hold space. • Communicate nonviolently. • Think systemically. • Maintain healthy boundaries within the family. • Recognize the impact of your own hidden emotional injuries from childhood.

Practice Radical Acceptance

In the early 1990s, psychologist Marsha Linehan explored the struggles that patients and their families have in accepting and coping with mental illnesses that are challenging to treat. Linehan (1993, 2020) understood the healing potential of radical acceptance in these families. Radical acceptance involves the capacity to accept a situation without judgment. It is important to stress that acceptance is not the same thing as approval or an excuse for unhealthy behaviors. It is the realization that you can't fight against reality; you can't go back in time no matter how hard you try. In Daniel's situation, it is the capacity for Arturo and his wife, Lucia, to view Daniel's situation from an unbiased observer perspective and to accept that their son's mental health disorder is out of their control. Radical acceptance does not ask you to disconnect from your feelings of sadness or loss but rather to embrace those emotions. Radical acceptance has also been described as the ability to acknowledge reality fully (Linehan, 2020).

Before you can practice radical acceptance, you will need to learn how to accept your adult child's mental health disorder as it exists without judging or wanting it to be different. This can be a difficult concept to wrap your head around, and it is essential to your role as wise counsel. To gain a better understanding of what this concept is, let's first see an example of what it is not. Parents often deny or minimize the seriousness of their young adult's mental health issue and Daniel's father is no different. Consider a story about Daniel and his father, told from the perspective of Lucia, which does not employ radical acceptance:

> It was about 11:00 a.m. on a Saturday and I was in the basement catching up on laundry and ironing from the week. All of a sudden, I heard this commotion coming from upstairs. Mostly, I heard Arturo yelling. His voice is so loud, and he doesn't realize how frightening he can be. I heard the sound of a door slamming. It sounded like it was coming from Daniel's room.

By the time I got up the stairs, Arturo was yelling at Daniel about not getting up earlier and going out and finding a job. He is always pestering Daniel about this, and I know Daniel is trying. It is tough out there. There are just not many jobs now for young people without a college degree. By the time I got to Daniel's room, I saw that Arturo had gone overboard. He actually poured water all over Daniel while he was lying in bed. I can't stand the yelling and cursing and the walking on eggshells. I begged Arturo to talk to his son calmly and reasonably. Instead, he just stomped out like he usually does when there is a conflict in the house. "I just can't deal with this right now," he shouted as he left.

For Daniel's father, Arturo, the sight of his son in bed late in the morning triggers an immediate and visceral response. He doesn't accept that Daniel is depressed and anxious and thinks "This isn't how things were supposed to go in my family." He feels stuck and frustrated that he cannot change Daniel. Arturo's aggressive reaction and his behavior only compound the underlying stress and turmoil in Daniel's family.

In many families, an adult child's diagnosis of a mental health disorder is often met with denial, avoidance, or fruitlessly wishing things were different. Like some parents, Arturo has difficulty not only accepting the reality of his son's depressive disorder but also that he can't do anything to change it. He believes that Daniel's symptoms are a ruse to get out of growing up and thinks that Daniel should be getting ready to head to the professional baseball league and not at home sleeping late. As long as these thoughts persist, he will be stuck in bitterness, anger, and sadness. It would be helpful for Arturo to be honest and courageous, and to admit to himself his concerns about Daniel's mental health disorder. Otherwise, tension and stress that come with fighting the reality of Daniel's depression can be immobilizing for Arturo.

Becoming a wise counsel does not happen overnight. It is important to acknowledge that this is a process that takes a lot of conscious effort and practice. As a parent, being educated about your adult child's illness goes hand in hand with your ability to develop radical acceptance. If Arturo learns about depression and familiarizes himself with various treatments and resources for Daniel, he likely may be able to move ahead on his journey. He may also learn a fundamental truth about parenting: "As much as I love Daniel, I can't keep him safe. I can't predict or control his future."

This experience of letting go can be likened to a swimmer's nightmare of being caught in a rip current. Do not try to swim directly to the shore because this will only zap your energy. Instead, swim parallel to the shoreline (Leatherman, 2003). For parents who are trying to come to grips with their young adult's mental illness, too much energy may be expended at times in trying to deny or rail against what they are seeing. That energy is better used in working to learn more about the mental illness and find ways to support their adult child while allowing them their autonomy. Radical acceptance is a tool to promote this shift in perspective that allows the parent to see reality for what it is. See Exhibit 7.2 for general guidelines to

---

EXHIBIT 7.2. Practice Radical Acceptance of Your Adult Child's Mental Health Issue

- **Notice**: When do I resist acknowledging my adult child's mental health issue?
- **Ask myself**: What feelings emerge when I am resisting?
- **Imagine this**: I accept my young adult's mental health disorder. How am I feeling now and what am I doing differently?
- **Let go**: Say to myself: "I can't control everything" and "I can only do my best to support my child."

help you begin to work toward radical acceptance of your young adults' mental health disorder.

Now let's look at a story that exemplifies Rachel's progress on her journey toward radical acceptance. The conversation below between Rachel and Jessie occurred after Jessie told her mom that she was definitely interested in scheduling a session with a therapist offering online therapy. Rachel felt relieved that Jessie planned to follow through on her recommendation to get help. Additionally, Jessie had a job interview scheduled for the next morning followed by lunch with her mom. Rachel was excited to have lunch with Jessie and to learn how her interview went. Rachel arrived at their favorite lunch place, sat at their special table, and waited and waited, but Jessie never showed. Let's listen as Rachel describes the conversation:

> The phone rang 5 or 6 times before Jessie answered in a groggy voice, "Hello?"
>
> "Jessie, are you okay? Why aren't you here?" I asked.
>
> "I overslept, Mom. I didn't hear the alarm, I guess." Her words were a bit slurred, and she seemed out of it. I wondered if she was hungover.
>
> "But what about your interview this morning?" I asked. As the conversation continued, I discovered that Jessie didn't go to her interview. She said she had a "bad day" yesterday. She had another panic attack and got very little sleep last night. Her alarm didn't go off for some reason. Jessie said she needed to hang up and call the contact person for the job to see if she could reschedule the interview.
>
> I was in shock. I felt like I was on an emotional roller coaster. I wanted to believe lately that Jessie was over the hump of her anxiety and was committed to getting help. Maybe I'm kidding myself; her alcohol and pot use may be worse than I thought. To think she slept through a job interview! The Jessie I raised always followed through on her commitments. This is not like her at all; she really was a responsible and conscientious kid.

Using Exhibit 7.2 as a guide, let's explore how Rachel might manage her own distress more effectively. Rachel may start by asking herself, "What am I feeling and thinking when I push back against the idea that my daughter has severe anxiety and may be misusing substances?" Rachel is likely feeling a mix of emotions including anger, hopelessness, sadness, frustration, and guilt. It's important for Rachel to acknowledge her feelings without judgment. She never expected her daughter to experience anxiety and to struggle emotionally. Rachel can't stop thinking that life is not supposed to be this way; it's simply not fair. More than anything, Rachel wants to take care of Jessie and to make sure she is okay. The problem is Jessie's mental health is not up to Rachel; she has no control over Jessie's decisions regarding treatment. Rachel has a choice. She can either continue to push back and get nowhere or she can consider the option of acceptance. If Rachel were to choose acceptance, she would acknowledge that Jessie's mental health (and other life situations) are outside of her control. To hold on to the illusion of control only intensifies Rachel's suffering and keeps her on the emotional roller coaster. Acceptance allows Rachel to let go and to focus on aspects of her own life where she can exert some control. Radical acceptance is a challenging process that takes time, patience, and lots of practice. This is difficult for a highly trained and competent EMT who is also a single mom and trying her best to keep her son and daughter on the right track.

Hold Space

Holding space (Plett, 2015, 2020) refers to the practice of intentionally being present for someone while listening attentively to what they have to say, even if the content of their message is difficult to hear. Holding space for your young adult means being fully present for as long as they need while simultaneously being aware of your own thoughts and feelings. It requires silence, empathy, and a withholding of judgment. Think of this space as being psychological as well as physical. It's important to note that it's possible to hold space for your young adult even if they live across the country rather than in close proximity. As a parent, this can be a difficult thing to do, regardless of where they are, because you want to share the wisdom of your experience to prevent them from making mistakes. You so want your young adult to do what you believe is best for them. And yet as a wise counsel you know they must make their own mistakes and learn from their missteps. Although difficult, holding space can be a meaningful gift to offer your young adult.

By practicing radical acceptance, Rachel is in a position to hold space for her daughter while Jessie figures out what to do. As her mother, Rachel can offer support and make suggestions when asked for advice; she cannot, however, make decisions for Jessie. It is important for Rachel to convey that she is present and ready to listen as Jessie takes the next steps.

Communicate Nonviolently

Parents who adopt a wise counsel role are able to communicate clearly and compassionately in families where there may be considerable stress and conflict. One tool we urge parents to include in their tote bag is nonviolent communication. This approach was developed by psychologist Marshall Rosenberg and is used in various fields including counseling, education, mediation, and organizational management. Rosenberg's (2015) approach recognized the potential for words to harm others and provides us with a framework for learning how to be more intentional and compassionate when we speak with others.

The practice of nonviolent communication requires that parents use many of the skills we covered in Chapter 2, such as listening intently, expressing empathy, and practicing the basics of effective communication. The ability to be aware of your feelings and to self-regulate emotions is an important prerequisite to the nonviolent communication process. This may be especially challenging for people who have grown up in families where the expression of feelings was discouraged or in families where feelings were expressed through yelling and screaming without respect for other family members. At times, emotions are mixed, and it may be difficult to tell what we are feeling. When communicating with others, we often make assumptions about what they are feeling, and we may blame them for how we feel.

The capacity to tune into your thoughts and recognize recurring thought patterns is also a prerequisite to the nonviolent communication process. As we discussed in Chapter 5, when we become familiar with our self-talk, we identify particular patterns of thoughts that are overly negative and rigid. We can practice distancing ourselves from our thoughts and thus keep them from influencing our behavior.

Finally, the nonviolent communication process demands being attuned to our own needs and being able to verbalize them to others. This may be the most challenging aspect of the nonviolent communication process for several reasons. In many families, children are socially conditioned in such a way as either to question their needs or not acknowledge them. The hesitancy to verbalize our needs to others can also stem from a prior history of relationships where our needs were either denied or addressed in an inconsistent manner. Some of us may hesitate because we fear being perceived by others as too "needy." Just as our culture discourages men from expressing feelings, women are often expected to recognize others' needs but at the same time to minimize their own.

The nonviolent communication process can be challenging. To illustrate how the process works, consider an example of the long-standing conflict between Pete and Ian over Ian's internet misuse. Pete has tried to discuss his concerns on several occasions, and the last time he and Ian talked, he felt as though they achieved a breakthrough. However, in the past few weeks, Ian has seemed to return to his old patterns of behavior. He is spending increasing amounts of time on the computer. At a recent family gathering with Pete's sister and brother-in-law, he observed Ian with his iPhone at brunch, seemingly oblivious to the conversation. This was the last straw for Pete. Pete knew from the past that his attempts to talk to Ian about his internet use usually resulted in his own anger growing as Ian became defensive and tried to minimize the problem. He waited until his anger subsided before approaching Ian.

Table 7.1 contains descriptions of each step along with an example of a statement that illustrates each step. As you can see from the examples in the table, Pete describes, in specific and neutral terms, the details of the situation that led to the present conflict. This is not an easy process, particularly because in many cases the current conflict has been a recurring one. One or both parties may have had previous conversations in the past, or possibly swept the issue under the rug.

Pete then describes how he felt about what happened, being careful to refrain from assigning blame to Ian for how he felt. Statements like "you made me mad" or "you hurt my feelings" will likely encourage Ian to respond defensively or not at all. It is important that Pete take ownership of what he is feeling.

The next step involves identifying the connection between what you are feeling and what you need. Unpleasant feelings usually result from unmet needs. In this case, Pete is upset because Ian didn't acknowledge his aunt and uncle during brunch, and often ignores his father when they are at home together.

TABLE 7.1. The Four-Step Nonviolent Communication Process

Step	Example
1. Observation: Staying as close to the facts versus using words that convey judgment and evaluation (e.g., right/wrong, good/bad)	"Yesterday during brunch with Aunt Theresa and Uncle Vince, I looked over at you several times and noticed you were texting on your cell."
2. Feelings: Using feeling words versus words that describe thoughts (self-talk, beliefs)	"I felt angry and embarrassed when I saw you texting while we were having brunch."
3. Needs: Using words that describe internally derived states versus describing preferences for specific behaviors that are directed at meeting needs	"I value our family time—especially when we aren't able to see Aunt Theresa and Uncle Vince very often because they live so far away. I would like you to understand and respect this."
4. Requests: Using specific and concrete words to describe what you want and avoiding vague language and "shoulds" (e.g., words that convey obligation or duty)	"How about we sit down and talk? I've got a hunch that you were uncomfortable. I want to understand what it was that may have triggered your need to pick up your phone and start texting during the meal."

The final step in the nonviolent communication process involves making requests. These must be doable—that is direct, present-oriented, and specific. These must also be phrased in positive terms, for example, asking for what you want versus what you don't want. It is helpful to state your needs and ask your young adult for a buy-in and consider your request.

Learning nonviolent communication is like learning a new language; it takes work and practice. We encourage you to begin by taking small steps; it is not easy to identify why we feel the way we do. It may be easier to practice what you want to say before sitting down with your emerging adult. Because communication is a two-way street, you may find yourself struggling to use the language of nonviolent communication with your adult child. In that case, the two of you may consider the possibility of seeking therapy or professional coaching to assist you both with this.

Think Systemically

Assuming the role of wise counsel involves, among other things, adopting a systems-oriented perspective. Systems thinking is currently used in many areas and work environments (e.g., businesses, health care settings, organizational management). In general, a systems approach is a lens that allows us to look at problems from a broader and more disciplined perspective and to appreciate all interconnections between factors that contribute to problems or conflicts. When we appreciate the broader perspective of things we tend not to blame others, and we react less impulsively.

For our purposes, a family is an example of a system. Every family develops its own organizational structure, boundaries, and rules. And therefore, each family system is unique and requires the presence of all family members to complete the family unit. Likewise, what happens to one family member will impact all other family members. So, to understand one family member, you need to understand the entire family unit.

Let's use the analogy of a mobile, dancing over a baby's crib, to capture the complexity of these dynamics in a family system. When a sudden wind hits one part of the mobile, it causes the other parts to spin around in an attempt to achieve balance. As one family member "bumps" against the other, it forces that person to adapt, sometimes in unhealthy ways.

Stressful events can upset the entire family system and disrupt well-established relationship patterns. In the case of Daniel's family, Arturo has been coping with the stress associated with Daniel's depression by isolating himself and using substances. There are many repercussions of Arturo's behavior, but the most obvious is his distancing from everyone in his family. As he isolates himself because of the anger and resentment he feels, Lucia focuses her attention on Daniel. From a different perspective, it can be argued that Arturo is disengaging in part due to his perception that Lucia is overly involved with Daniel. The more Lucia focuses on Daniel, the more isolated and alone his sister Elena feels. She copes with her invisibility within the family by escaping to her friend's house where she feels comfortable and protected from the stress of home. You can see how the behavior of one member affects all the members of the family. It is not surprising, then, that Daniel's depression and anxiety caused reverberations throughout his family. No member of the family remains untouched by the presence of mental illness in the family.

Underfunctioning and Overfunctioning

In our relationships, one person's actions are linked to another person's actions. In other words, when one family member steps in and *overfunctions*—that is, does too much work and takes on too many responsibilities within the family—it often leads another member to *underfunction*, or withdraw. For example, your spouse is a "neat-nik" and has been through much of your relationship, and you notice that you have gradually become less and less involved in the household. You even have occasionally said to your spouse, "Why should I bother to help? You always tell me I don't do it right."

Let's consider another example from one of our families. Lucia and Arturo have bickered over Daniel and the best way to handle him and his depression. When Daniel left school and came home, Arturo read him the riot act. He told Daniel he needed to get a job right away and to pay for room and board. Arturo threatened to take Daniel's car away if he didn't get a job. Daniel did get a job at a restaurant, but he was let go after 9 months due to the COVID pandemic.

A typical argument between Lucia and Arturo goes something like this:

> *Lucia:* Why are you so hard on Daniel, Arturo? He is struggling right now, and you just keep yelling at him to snap out of it. Why can't you be gentler with him and try to understand him? I keep having to console him after you get so angry.
>
> *Arturo:* You coddle him too much. You always have. You had to go and mess with his schooling by getting that medical withdrawal. Look at him, Lucia. He's nothing but a lump in his bed. It does no good for me to say anything. That's why I just throw my hands up and walk away.

It is easy to imagine how these ways of relating to each other become more rigid over time. Each partner retreats to their corner and repeats the same behavior again and again, and nothing changes. Watch what happens when we take this same situation and view it through a systemic lens. We are taking a step back and broadening our perspective. When we do this, we are able to be more objective and have less need to blame someone or something. When we don't take that broader perspective, we get stuck.

ENDING THE BLAME GAME

Arturo gets angry because he thinks Daniel spends too much time in his room on the computer. Arturo loses his temper with his son and lashes out at him with complaints about not finding another job and not contributing to household expenses, staying up too late and sleeping too long in the mornings. In other words, it appears that Arturo is blaming Daniel for the depression. As a result, he is angry with his son.

Arturo is engaged in the blame game, which serves no useful purpose. Instead, systemic thinking allows us to shift from a linear cause and effect manner of thinking. We can consider a broad range of factors that may contribute to Daniel's oversleeping and lack of motivation as well as his depressed mood. It would help Arturo to look at his situation in a different way and understand there are many reasons for Daniel's behavior.

ADDITIONAL FACTORS IN SYSTEMIC THINKING

As a wise counsel, it is essential for you to understand that in addition to viewing your family dynamics through a systemic lens, you must also consider the fact that your sociocultural contexts are actually complex systems. Sociocultural factors such as race, ethnicity, immigrant status, religious affiliation, socioeconomic level, gender identity, sexual orientation, disability, and so on impact the ways in which you define yourself individually and as part of a family unit. Each part of your identity is vulnerable to some form of discrimination or mistreatment. Your ability to recognize this and to understand how it impacts your life and your opportunities is crucial. In your role as wise counsel, you will need to have a firm grasp of how the multiple systems in which you live impact your life and your young adult's life for better and worse so that you can support their journey toward autonomy. The impact of sociocultural factors on psychological distress and access to mental health treatment cannot be overemphasized.

For example, a person living from paycheck to paycheck may struggle to find adequate mental health care for their young adult given the limited range of treatment options. They may or may not have health care coverage, and if they do, it may or may not cover mental health services. Already living under a heavy burden of stress, this could push a parent to the brink.

MAINTAIN HEALTHY BOUNDARIES WITHIN THE FAMILY

In Chapter 2, we stressed the importance of setting and maintaining healthy individual boundaries. We now turn to a discussion of boundaries in a family system. Just as the individual with weak boundaries cannot function effectively as a person, so too families with weak boundaries do not function effectively. Because there is little or no emotional separation between family members, everyone winds up overreaching and getting into the other family members' "stuff." In psychology, this is known as being *enmeshed*, which makes it difficult, if not impossible, to sort out who I am, separate and apart from who you are. The young adult who pursues a career and or a life partner based on what would make their parents happy has likely not been able to separate themselves emotionally from the parents or to consider what they need in their own life.

To help us better understand the concept of enmeshed boundaries from a parental perspective, let's imagine that your son received a failing grade on a chemistry test, or your daughter was fired by her boss for "no reason." In these instances, unbeknownst to your young adult, you fire off an email to the professor or march into the workplace to have it out with your daughter's boss almost as if it was you who was fired. In each instance, you are disrespecting your young adult and, by default, questioning their ability to handle their situation on their own. Parents in such situations intrude into their young adult's life, hindering the ability of the young person to undertake the necessary steps of learning to function autonomously in their life.

Likewise, families with very rigid boundaries are disconnected from one another on an emotional and physical level. The young adult has little or no input from family, and no one is there to help them think through their decisions and make course corrections when necessary. They also struggle in interpersonal relationships, not having had the modeling from parents on how to engage in healthy ways with others.

Families with healthy boundaries respect the privacy of other family members and are flexible in their dealings with each other. Parents may offer input as they see potential red flags. There is give and take with the young adult, who is allowed to grow and develop their own interests and explore their individual pathway without having to drag the whole family along with them. It's all part of the process of becoming a wise counsel.

We do need to say a word about boundaries and culture because the definition of boundaries may be quite different depending on the cultural context. Some cultures value intergenerational closeness such as daily contact with adult children. This does not mean such families have enmeshed boundaries but rather that they structure family relationships in a different way than our western culture. With Lucia, what appears to be helicopter behavior may actually be an acceptable way to deal with her son based on her Guatemalan cultural background and learning. We want to be careful not to assign the norms of our own culture to families whose cultural norms are different.

We learn from our own families of origin about how to construct boundaries within a family, and Daniel's parents are no different. Their experiences in their own families served as important lessons in how they would interact with their own children. A parent's capacity to set and maintain healthy family boundaries with their adult children is, in large measure, dependent on being aware of their own feelings and thoughts. They must also keep in mind that their family is changing, and their adult child has a life of their own.

 ## RECOGNIZE THE IMPACT OF YOUR OWN HIDDEN EMOTIONAL INJURIES FROM CHILDHOOD

In Chapter 4, we discussed the significant role of *adverse childhood events*, or childhood trauma in the development of adult depression and anxiety disorders. Many people associate the word *trauma* with sexual or physical abuse and neglect and don't relate to the idea of having experienced an injury of a different sort in their own childhood. It may be more helpful to suggest that while our childhoods were generally positive, we may have also experienced stressful, negative events that taxed our childhood abilities to cope. Some examples might include having a learning problem or disability as a child that was never recognized or addressed or having a childhood illness that required painful medical procedures and periods of separation from family members. You may have grown up with several siblings in a family with few economic resources, and as a result, your parents were often preoccupied and inattentive to your needs. Whatever the particular event, as a child you may have felt lonely, afraid, and a sense of shame. We don't always know the feelings are there but they have a tendency to leak out, particularly during times of stress.

In Arturo's case, his childhood memories include being shamed and ridiculed by his father (Daniel's grandfather) for having feelings of vulnerability, fear, and sadness. From the perspective of family systems, Arturo's painful childhood experiences served as a template for his interactions with his own family. Arturo responded to Daniel's symptoms of depression and anxiety with anger and controlling behaviors like his father. Arturo learned to internalize feelings of vulnerability—and later, to numb these through alcohol use. As we discussed in Chapter 3, one common strategy people use to avoid painful feelings is through overuse of alcohol and drugs, overindulging in junk food, bingeing on Netflix, scrolling mindlessly on social media, and so on. These are short-term fixes and are likely to result in these feelings resurfacing and becoming even stronger.

For another perspective, let's revisit Claire as she discusses her recent realization about her childhood:

> When Anne's doctor told me that he thought she had bipolar disorder I was devastated. These are words I never wanted to hear. When I was a little girl, I remember my maternal grandfather yelling at my grandma while he threw things around in the kitchen. He acted like he was crazy. When he wasn't acting crazy, he laid on the couch all day. There were also times when he disappeared for weeks at a time. My mom and grandma used to whisper about him when they thought I couldn't hear them. They said he was mentally ill. When I was older, I put it all together. He had bipolar disorder.
>
> Did I pass these genes down to Anne? Is her mental illness because of me? Realistically I can tell myself that it is not my fault. But my heart is not there yet. I have no idea what to do. Anne's father listens, but he never has much to say. I'm not sure what to do with all these feelings. I wonder if counseling might help, but the idea of talking to a stranger . . . I just don't know if I'm comfortable with that.

Learning how to heal from these childhood injuries takes time and energy, and when your young adult is suffering, time and energy may feel in short supply. Yet talking with a trusted friend, partner, or clergy member who is able to sit with you and acknowledge your pain can be a source of healing. It is not uncommon for people like Claire to be hesitant to speak with a "stranger" or therapist. However, there is value in talking with someone who is outside your situation and is trained to listen without giving advice, wishing away the pain, or denying the experience. To be there for your young adult when they are struggling, it is important to be able to recognize your own difficulties and emotional baggage from childhood.

Claire's situation illustrates the importance of being honest with family about the skeletons that may be hiding out in your closets. For most of us, being transparent with medical issues such as cancer or diabetes in the family is a way to help alert family members to potential health risks. However, when it comes to mental health issues, families tend to follow the double standard of keeping these concerns a secret. Such a practice can result in a situation similar to Claire's where the family secret from two generations back is creating significant and unnecessary distress. As wise counsel, this honesty with yourself and your family is often a difficult task, but it is an essential part of healing and moving forward.

SUMMARY

In this chapter we encouraged you to consider pivoting to the role of wise counsel, which expands on the skills associated with the advanced coach role. When parents of adult children assume a wise counsel role, they practice radical acceptance, hold space for their young adult, and communicate in a nonviolent manner with them in potentially volatile or high-conflict contexts. They think systemically—that is, they understand the impact of the mental health issue on the entire family and do what is necessary to maintain healthy family boundaries. Furthermore, they recognize that at times their adult children's symptoms and behaviors may be triggers for their own long buried memories of emotional injury. This can feel unsettling to the parent as they interact with their adult children. Being able to recognize the impact of one's own hidden emotional stuff from childhood helps the parent to understand more clearly where their current feelings may be coming from and not get tangled up with their adult child's situation.

Now that you are fully immersed in the role of wise counsel, it will be to your advantage to understand and process the many losses you have experienced and continue to experience on your journey with your young adult. Coupled with that is a deeper level of skill regarding your own self-care. While we have periodically addressed these themes, we firmly believe that their importance is such that they deserve their own chapters. In Chapter 8, we focus on ways to recognize and mourn your losses, and in Chapter 9, we further embrace the need for self-care and self-compassion.

POINTS TO POCKET

- Knowledge + experience = good judgment. Or as journalist and musician Miles Kington is often attributed to have said, "Knowledge is knowing that a tomato is a fruit. Wisdom is not putting it in a fruit salad."
- Listen up: Radical acceptance allows you to stop struggling and begin to see your young adult's mental health disorder for what it really is instead of how you would like it to be.
- Think systemically: Systems thinking takes us away from a laser-focused, quick-fix mentality and allows us to see the big picture, be more self-reflective, and avoid the blame game.

- Words have power: Nonviolent communication allows us to be more intentional and compassionate when we talk with our young adults and other family members.
- Know yourself: Whether we like it or not, our childhood experiences impact the way we see ourselves and how we interact with others.

III

RIGHT SIDE UP AGAIN

CHAPTER 8

MOURNING YOUR LOSSES

Although the world is full of suffering, it is full also of the overcoming of it.

—Helen Keller

"Tears and fears and feeling proud," the iconic words to "Both Sides Now" sung by Joni Mitchell (1969) appear to fit the rhythm of parenting for many of us. By the time your young adult reaches adult status, you have truly seen life from both sides, up and down, win and lose. And somehow you are still standing. Your parenting journey has involved many pivots, transitions, and losses both large and small. Loss is a part of life, and the older we get, the more losses we experience.

In this chapter, we invite you to really engage that skill of educating yourself as we explore the experience of loss from various perspectives. When we say "loss," we mean a wide range of situations you may be experiencing. Many times, we hear the words "loss" and "grief" and immediately think of a loved one's death. This is certainly one type of loss. However, the most common types of loss for parents of young adults are nondeath losses. For example, some parents have difficulty coming to terms with the fact that their little boy or little girl has grown up. They struggle with the fact that those childhood years they enjoyed with their offspring are now over. Many other parents are grieving as they come to terms with the fact that their adult child has a mental health disorder. These parents never imagined their adult child would be in so much distress that they could not stay in school, maintain a job, or live independently. These parents are feeling an acute loss of the idealized vision of parenthood that has not come to fruition. Although their emerging adult will likely get better, especially if they get professional help, this is still a tough loss for the parents.

We open with a discussion of the assumptive world that each of us has created over time to provide a sense of security and control. We next present a continuum of losses including necessary loss, temporary loss, living/nondeath loss, and finality loss. We discuss the variation in support that often accompanies different types of loss, including the degree of connection to others or isolation parents feel following the loss. We unpack grief, the process of handling our losses, and the task of meaning-making as we continue to live our lives. In addition, we look at permanent loss including nondeath conditions (e.g., loss of vision resulting in blindness or paralysis from a spinal cord injury); accidental deaths, which sadly are common in the young adult cohort; and the loss of a young adult by suicide.

It is important to understand that although loss and grief are universal experiences, we each move through them in our own unique way. Even when all members of a family experience the same loss, each person may interpret and deal with that loss differently. There is no right way to do grief and no magic timetable for when it will end. We will also provide an additional tool or two for your tote bag.

ASSUMPTIVE WORLD

Let's begin our discussion of loss by considering first the term *assumptive world* (Parkes, 1988), which clinicians typically use to talk about traumatic loss. For our purposes here, we employ the term as a framework for understanding the impact of losses of many kinds.

Our assumptive worlds are the beliefs that ground us and help us to feel safe; they allow us to believe that there is a future (Kauffman, 2002). Such beliefs are deeply ingrained and develop through our experiences of attachment and within the context of our culture. Over time, the assumptive world provides a sense of security as we move about in our lives. The assumptive world is made up of three parts (Janoff-Bulman, 1989; see Exhibit 8.1):

1. Our belief about the world—the extent to which we see the world as good and people as being trustworthy.
2. Our belief about how things should work—our view of the world as having meaning and being predictable, or not ("if I work hard, I will be rewarded").
3. Our belief about ourselves—our view of ourselves as being okay and up to the challenges we face, or not ("I am a worthy, competent being").

Based on our past experiences, we think we know what to expect in the current situation. If we see ourselves as capable and confident that we can handle things, the door to the future is open. This belief system guides us throughout the day almost as if on auto-pilot, and we have little need to challenge it.

For those who are less than positive about the goodness and predictability of the world, and their ability to cope, their belief system and assumptive world are going to be different. Rather than

---

EXHIBIT 8.1. A Positive Assumptive World

- Belief that the world is good.
- Belief that the world is predictable and has meaning.
- Belief in the self as capable and worthy.

lending itself to a strong foundation on which to proceed, their negative mindset leaves them with a diminished sense of order and safety as well as doubts about their own worth and ability to handle what comes their way.

For our parents, Claire and Stan with Anne's bipolar I diagnosis, Arturo and Lucia with their son's depression and suicidal thoughts, Rachel confronting Jessie's acute anxiety symptoms, and Pete's struggle with his son's nonstop internet use, their assumptive worlds have taken a hit. For each of the parents, their own sense of their ability to cope and the safety and "goodness" of the world is going to determine their response to the situations with which they are faced. Each one's unique belief structures coupled with how they perceive the loss they are facing will determine how they fare. Regardless, experiencing a loss can begin to erode our beliefs and, depending on the nature of the loss, our assumptive world can be knocked right off its foundation. As we continue to move through the continuum of losses, we will explore in more detail how our assumptive worlds can be affected.

THE LOSS CONTINUUM

Using our continuum once again, keep in mind that losses vary greatly in their intensity and permanence. We urge you to keep this continuum of loss in mind as you continue reading. Also remember that not all losses at any point on the continuum are equally benign or heart wrenching for everyone. Using the loss continuum in Figure 8.1 as a guide, let's examine the experience of loss.

Necessary Loss

At the far left of the continuum are the *necessary losses* we all face as parents as our children grow. These begin in the weeks and months

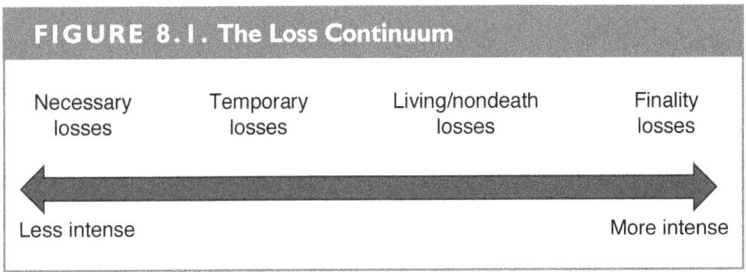

FIGURE 8.1. The Loss Continuum

| Necessary losses | Temporary losses | Living/nondeath losses | Finality losses |

Less intense   More intense

after a child comes into your life as you watch them grow and change. In Chapter 2, we talked about the pivot from caretaker to coach as your child turned 18 and became an adult according to the law. You had many chances to experience a loosening of your hold on your child, such as their first day of school, the first sleepover at a friend's house, perhaps their first sleepaway camp experience, and so on. Nevertheless, change is not always easy, and for many folks, it is something to be feared. This fear inhibits our ability to adapt and grow with the changing situation. Many losses are countered by joy, such as watching our little ones step up on the school bus or into the classroom for their first day of kindergarten. We are full of pride even as our eyes fill with tears. A page turns, a new chapter of their lives, and ours, begins.

There is, however, something unique in your child becoming a legal adult that sets a different tone for many in a parenting role. For some parents, this is an easy pivot as they step back, take a breath, and watch the launch. For others, however, it is much more difficult, especially if they have defined themselves by the role of caretaker. Regardless, it is another pivot we must contend with. The feeling of loss in these experiences is what we consider *necessary losses* on our continuum. They are necessary so that both our young adults and we, ourselves, can continue to grow. We don't want to minimize how hard these necessary losses can be for some folks; at the same time, we emphasize that such losses are a normal part of our lives.

Likewise, pivoting from coach or advanced coach to wise counsel involves another shift of your role as a parent and pulling back yet again from the teaching work of the coach to an advisory role with your young adult. For those of you still embodying the caretaker persona, this shift may seem huge and feel like you are losing another sphere of influence in your child's life. We want to assure you that you are not alone in feeling this way and the wise counsel pivot is necessary for you as a parent of a young adult.

Temporary Loss

Temporary losses are setbacks or those losses that usually have a relatively short-term impact on your life (e.g., a delay in getting your degree due to financial issues, or coming down with a serious, but not life-threatening, illness that forces you out of work for several months). If your young adult takes a semester off from school to figure out what they want to do, you may experience this as a loss and worry that they will not return. They sign up for classes for the next year with a renewed sense of what they want to study, and you breathe a sigh of relief. Or your adult child loses their job due to the employer going out of business. They have to move home because they can't afford their current living arrangements, and the freedom you had is now diminished due to their presence in your home. After 5 months, they find a new job, move out and again, a sigh of relief escapes as you regain your sense of freedom. In such situations, your assumptive world may shudder a bit, but it basically remains intact.

Living or Nondeath Loss

Living loss is a descriptor for many kinds of losses we experience and must learn to live with over the long haul. Sometimes called nonfinite losses, these reflect the kind of loss that seemingly has no end. No one died, but you experienced the loss of a cherished goal, or idea, or something you believed would happen but didn't. In other words, this is the loss of what will never be. Living loss involves living in a changed world, such as an adult child with a mental health issue who no longer seems to be the person they once were. And there are reminders of the loss every day. For example, you and your partner are planning for the eventual launch of your last child from college to a real job. Freedom is within sight and so is that trip you've been talking about for several years. And then your partner has a stroke and requires your constant care and daily assistance to manage basic life tasks. Not only is the trip no longer possible, but the future you had dreamed of together is derailed. Your partner's debilitation is a tangible and constant reminder of what you have lost.

Another example of living loss occurs if your emerging adult develops a chronic physical health problem or a mental health disorder that sidelines them from the mainstream activities of a typical young adult. The plan or dream you had for them is no longer doable, and the loss can be significant for you. Your assumptions about the world being a benevolent place, orderly and meaningful, are shaken, and you may engage in self-blame for what your adult child is going through. You may wonder, "How could I let this happen?" Well, you didn't. Life intervenes in our plans at times, taking us on a different path than the one we thought we were traveling. Making sense of such living losses is essential; this involves reworking our assumptive world to incorporate the loss and reestablish a sense of equilibrium. It also involves creating a new sense of meaning for ourselves and our own lives, often without the support of the community around us. We'll say more about meaning in just a minute.

Claire and Stan came face-to-face with their own living loss when Anne was diagnosed with bipolar I disorder. Anne was no longer the daughter they knew, and the future was now uncertain. Claire and Stan had so many questions, and their loss was tangible.

> Where has our daughter gone? Where is that sweet child who used to sing and dance around the house and pound the piano with gusto? She was so smart and so talented! She was going to be a wildlife biologist and travel the world studying animals in their natural habitats. How could this happen? How did we get to this point? We were really a close-knit family—not perfect, but we worked. We don't deserve this! What do we do now?

Claire and Stan are feeling what many of us could feel in this situation. The future has taken an unanticipated turn, and the safety of their assumptive worlds has been shaken. They are anxious and afraid for Anne and feel helpless as to what to do next. We talk a lot about resilience in Chapter 9. However, it is important to stress here that the level of resilience within Claire and Stan will, to a large extent, determine how they handle the changed world in which they now live. Their ability, both individually and as a couple, to adapt and meet the current moment will help them navigate the storm with more confidence.

We can also look at Arturo's strong belief that Daniel will become a major league baseball player. He has fixed this dream for his son in his mind and now must face the very real possibility that this dream will not be realized. Coming to grips with this loss will be difficult for Arturo. His assumptive world has been rocked and, just like with Claire and Stan, Arturo's level of resilience and his ability to shift with the circumstances will determine how he is able to weather the current storm.

Living losses can and do involve the upending of family stability due to the challenges your young adult is facing. If you recall from Chapter 7 our discussion about family systems and the skill of "thinking systemically," you will remember how one family member's emotional distress reverberates throughout the entire family. Their emotional distress quite often changes the way family dynamics flow and how family members interact with each other. For example, if you as a parent are putting much of your time and effort into trying to help your adult child find mental health services, or perhaps just focusing on what to do next, you have diverted time and attention from your partner and other children. You may find yourself being short with one of your other children, telling them you don't have time for this or that, or simply forget to show up for an activity you had promised to attend. Likewise, snapping at your partner or declining to engage in conversation with them because you have too much on your mind, are ways of signaling that something is out of balance. Family stability can be rocky in these circumstances, and this is a loss for all of you. The ground under each of your assumptive worlds may be getting a bit squishy!

Finality Loss

At the far right of the continuum, we use the term *finality loss* meaning the loss is final and often traumatic. Some such losses may also be living losses. For example, when a person loses a function, such as the ability to see or walk, these are permanent changes in their life. They continue to live, but the loss doesn't change. The loss is irreversible, and the impact often reverberates for years or, in the case of mobility or function loss, perhaps for the rest of one's life.

The loss of a loved one through death is what we typically think of when we think of a final loss. It is permanent, and we must figure out how to continue without that loved one in our life. Let's move to a discussion of accidental death, suicidal thoughts and behaviors, and loss by suicide.

Accidental Death

One type of finality loss particularly prevalent in the young adult population is that of accidental death. This age group is populated with risk takers and young people willing to push the boundaries of what we might consider safe behaviors. Experimenting with drugs and alcohol, driving a car or boat while under the influence, or jumping their mountain bike across a ravine on a dare are examples of what young adults might do to test their limits. When we couple such behaviors with the fact that their prefrontal cortexes are not yet fully formed, we have potentially dangerous activities and inadequate judgment to know when to apply the brakes. This results in serious and often permanent injury or in death. Parents in such instances are vulnerable to complicated or prolonged grief, which we will talk about shortly.

Let's take the instance of a young woman who recently turned 21. For her birthday, her parents gifted her an older, but still rather classy, sports sedan. She is thrilled and collects some friends for a road trip to a lakeside cabin in the New Hampshire mountains for the weekend. Soon some of their guy friends show up with beer, and they are all gathered around a beach fire at the edge of the water. Eventually, the birthday girl, having consumed five or six beers, decides it's time for a swim, and heads barefoot down to the dock. As she takes off at a sprint for the end of the dock, her feet slip on the dewy wet boards, she loses her balance and falls off the edge of the dock striking her head on a metal cleat. Someone at the fire circle yells "splash!" They wait for their friend to pop up, but the water is still. One of the young women runs down to the dock looking for the missing friend. She screams for someone to call 911 and jumps into the water to search for her friend. It is several hours before the parents are notified that their daughter is dead of what looks to be an accidental drowning.

Other instances of accidental death occur due to violence. Whether being at the wrong place at the wrong time when a violent act occurs, such as a shooting at a university, workplace, or community social gathering, random violence can leave loved ones dealing with the loss of their young adult with no answers to the question of "why?" and a difficult road ahead. Regardless of the type of accidental loss, parents and other loved ones are left with the horrible reality that this death didn't have to occur, and that can make grieving the loss that much more difficult and drawn out.

A parent can be wracked with guilt for "letting" their adult child attend the outdoor concert, participate in extreme mountain biking, or giving them the car that led them to their untimely death. In reality, the adult child made the decision to go to the concert, play the sport, or drive with friends to the lake. They are legally adults and don't require permission. Even if Mom or Dad bought the mountain bike on which their son tried to jump the ravine, the son still made the decision to take that risk. The young woman in the preceding example made the decision to take her friends to the lake, drink to excess, and go for a swim with too much alcohol in her system. Uncoupling the parent's responsibility from the tragic death is indeed a difficult challenge, and a necessary one for the parent to face. It also may prevent the parent from having to experience prolonged grief, which we will get to in a minute.

 SUICIDAL THOUGHTS AND BEHAVIORS

As we mentioned in Chapter 4, emerging adults are a population at risk for suicide. Many will have suicidal ideation, or thoughts but never go any further than the thought. Others may make an attempt, or multiple attempts, and then move past the depression to have rich and full lives. And sadly, some young adults will carry out a lethal action to end their lives. Still others will be tormented by the thoughts for years.

When a young adult sends messages, subtle or otherwise, that their lives are just too difficult to handle anymore, parents naturally freak out, although their responses may look very different. Some will try to coax their adult child into believing it really isn't that bad and to look on the bright side. Others might blame the child for causing them pain, saying, "Why are you doing this to me? I don't deserve this." Still others may panic and rush their young adult to the emergency room. If you were a hoverer (think "helicopter parent") before, you may find yourself not wanting to let your young adult out of your sight. And there are also those parents who become enraged with their adult child, saying, "No son of mine is going to do this. Man up! Life is hard." This reaction is likely covering up the fact that the parent is terrified and feels a very real loss of control over the situation. Regardless of the reaction, the parent's assumptive world is shaken, and their life is forever changed.

Let's look at Arturo's situation again:

> My son was back at school, and I thought things were going better. Then we have a knock on the door at midnight: It's a policewoman informing us that they received a call from Daniel's ex-girlfriend, Alessandra. She told the 911 operator that Daniel just texted her saying he doesn't want to live anymore and had just taken a bunch of pills. The police got to his apartment and found him semiconscious. He was in the ER at that moment. My wife and I got dressed quickly and rushed to the hospital. When we got to the bed where he was lying with a sheet pulled up to his waist, I lost it. I proceeded to unload on my son.
>
> "What are you doing? No son of mine does this! You have to be tough; you are a man! How dare you pull this sh*t?"
>
> I was so angry at him! I couldn't hold back! Meanwhile, Lucia collapsed in a puddle of tears.

The bottom line is that parents are frightened when their young adult talks about or tries to harm themselves. Arturo is no different. He is covering the fear with his anger, and this fear is what is driving his emotional outburst. His assumptive world has been severely shaken. As we said in the beginning of the book, the one thing most of us can agree on is that we want the best for our children. And this includes a safe passage to adulthood and beyond. When your adult child talks or acts in ways that suggest they may intentionally harm themselves, as Daniel did in this example, you can't help but have strong reactions. There may also be a sense of betrayal that is harder to acknowledge—the feeling of "how dare you say this, or do this, after all I've done for you," which shuts down your ability to deal with your child in a positive way. You love them dearly, and the idea of being "double-crossed" after all your efforts can be very real. You may also question your relationship with your young adult and wonder "Why couldn't you come to me if you were feeling this way?"

Your young adult seems to have taken direct aim at your sense of competence as a parent. And the world does not seem to be such a benign place anymore, does it? It certainly isn't the predictable place it appeared to be once upon a time. Your assumptive world feels pretty fragile right now as you confront the reality that your adult child is in danger.

Loss by Suicide

The loss of a young adult by suicide is perhaps the most horrific experience that any parent can have. Hands down, your assumptive world is blown off its foundation and you reel from the explosion of your "normal" life. For you that life no longer exists. One of the most common things for a parent to do following a death by suicide of their child is ask why. "Why did they choose to do this?" Parents are desperately searching for meaning in an act that seems so extreme. Close on the heels of asking "why?" is the strong tendency to engage in a lot of self-blame. How could I have let this happen to my adult child? How come I didn't see the signs? Sometimes parents externalize their anger into blaming others, (e.g., their own partner, their young adult's girlfriend or boyfriend, or another person). This is a prime example of when complicated or prolonged grief is likely to occur as the parents struggle to remain upright in a world that has fallen apart. We will talk about prolonged grief in just a minute.

Using the lens of thinking systemically introduced in Chapter 7, we can understand how the shock and emotional turmoil reverberate through the family. Each member struggles to make sense of what has happened and to find a path forward. Family dynamics often shift in the wake of a young adult's death by suicide. For example, parents may withdraw from each other or pull back from any interactions with other family members. Siblings may also withdraw, or they may attempt to fill their own and the lost sibling's shoes through academic pursuits. They may try to be the "fixer" in the family, working to keep the peace and not make any waves. In doing so, they run the risk of shortchanging their own goals and dreams. Parents may also push the sibling to "excel for two." At any rate, the shift in family dynamics can be tricky and unhealthy for all involved.

Coupled with guilt the parents might feel is the stigma associated with a death by suicide. A culture of silence surrounds the act itself and the family members who are devastated in its aftermath. This stigma is born in part from fear of what others will say when they hear about the death by suicide. Families may attempt to hide the circumstances of the death by saying in the obituary the person died unexpectedly at home. They may hesitate to talk about their loss with people outside the immediate circle of family and close friends who know what happened. As parents use secrecy to cope with the stigma they are feeling, there are negative consequences for their own mental well-being (Oexle et al., 2020).

Some people turn away from encounters with the bereaved family members because they don't know what to say or are afraid that anything they do say will be another dagger of pain for the grieving family. Whispers and quick changes in topic when a family member enters the room accompany the discomfort everyone is feeling and serve to isolate the grieving family members further from those who could possibly offer support. Because there is no open, honest conversation and opportunity to share feelings, the grieving process gets short-circuited.

For parents, there is a real sense that the world does not want to acknowledge their experience. A door slams shut at the first mention of suicide. They are living in a cone of silence, isolated from the rest of the community. If their adult child had terminal cancer, that door would be open. This great silence around suicide in our culture is something that inhibits the healing process for families. When the need for support is greatest, the support too often is lacking. Combined with the parents' perception that others are judging and even blaming them, the lack of support makes healing that much more difficult. As a parent, the loss of a young adult through suicide is a profound grief experience, one that will take time and much support to process. It is crucial that you take care of yourself in this process as you come to terms with the explosion of your assumptive world and work to reestablish your sense of well-being. We encourage you to seek help from a professional or consider attending a support group for survivors of suicide. We suggest the American Foundation for Suicide Prevention website (https://afsp.org/find-a-support-group) as a place to seek out group support. Individual therapy and support groups provide a forum for us to experience our loss in a safe environment. Let us turn now to a fuller understanding of what the work of grief is all about.

THE WORK OF GRIEF

Grief is our emotional response to a loss. It is a universal experience that we all feel at different times in our lives, and each of us experiences grief in our own unique way. Grief is what we feel inside. Bereavement and mourning are what we do to handle the loss (D. Kessler, 2019). It's important to understand that grief accompanies all kinds of loss, not just a loss through death. Thus, when your young adult is in psychological distress or struggling with a mental health disorder, grief is a natural response to the loss of that child you knew before the mental illness descended.

The process of adaptation and its companion, coping, come into play as we grieve. Adaptation is something that naturally evolves when we face significant change in our lives. This happens over time as we find a path forward. Coping refers to how we handle the pain and stress of the loss—the things we do to manage in the shorter term as we move through the adaptation process (Center for Prolonged Grief, n.d.).

You might wonder, "How long is too long to mourn?" We have already said there is no timetable for grief, and each of us does this work in our own time. Gradually, we move from having the loss on center stage in our daily life, to getting it out of our central focus and into a different place where it is still with us but doesn't occupy most of our waking hours. We don't forget it, but we find a path beyond it. This type of grief falls on one end of a continuum (see Figure 8.2) and has been called *normative* or *common grief*. At the other end of our continuum is *prolonged grief*, which we talk about shortly.

Normative or common grief initially involves a period of more intense mourning or acute grief. With acute or early grief, we often experience shock, numbness, a denial of the reality of our loss, as well

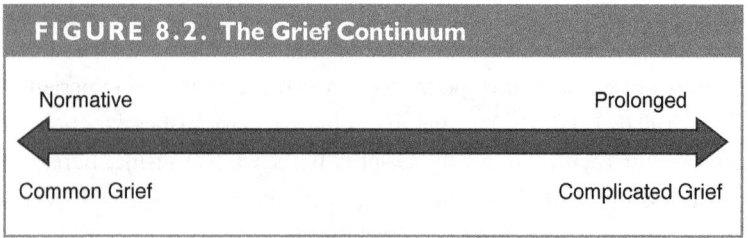

FIGURE 8.2. The Grief Continuum

Normative   Prolonged

Common Grief   Complicated Grief

as overwhelming sadness. The intensity of our acute grief will vary depending on the type of loss and may be influenced by both our culture and religious beliefs (Szuhany et al., 2021). Over time, we are able to integrate the loss and sadness and begin to reengage with our lives and relationships with others (A. H. Jordan & Litz, 2014). In other words, we are adapting to the loss.

Approximately 7% to 10% of the time, however, this adaptation process is interrupted (Szuhany et al., 2021). For folks in this category, the intense pain and sense of loss do not gradually diminish, and they are not able to move it off center stage after a year. This is called complicated or prolonged grief, where the person is not able to find the off-ramp from their grief. Prolonged grief, as it is more often called, can happen to anyone, but it is often associated with losing someone close to you suddenly in an accidental, inexplicable, or violent manner. Such deaths are senseless and have no satisfactory explanation for the question of "Why did this happen?" In addition, individuals who have a history of anxiety or mood disorders, such as depression, struggle with handling difficult emotions and lack social support, so are more vulnerable to experiencing prolonged grief (Szuhany et al., 2021). Hallmarks of prolonged grief include mourning that lasts more than a year for adults. This is accompanied by the presence of either an unremitting longing for the deceased person or a preoccupation with thoughts of the deceased individual.

For a formal diagnosis, an individual must exhibit at least three of the symptoms of prolonged grief (see Exhibit 8.2) daily for at least a month (Prigerson et al., 2022). They also must display an inability to reconnect with their previous existence or handle the basic fundamentals of daily life (taking care of themselves and their health, engaging in work and/or family responsibilities, etc.) during the year since the death occurred (American Psychiatric Association, 2022).

Let's consider how parents who experience the accidental death of a young adult might be vulnerable to prolonged grief.

EXHIBIT 8.2. Symptoms of Prolonged Grief

- Disruption in identity
- Denial that the death occurred
- Avoiding reminders that the person has died
- Unremitting emotional pain
- Struggle to reconnect with relationships and daily activities
- Feelings of emotional numbness
- Feeling life has no meaning since the death
- Extreme loneliness after the death

Returning to the example of the young woman who accidentally drowned while celebrating with her friends, her parents quite naturally reel from the shock of hearing that their daughter is dead. They are heartbroken and consumed with their grief, as well as the "if only" thoughts—"If only we hadn't given her the car, if only she hadn't been drinking, if only her friends could've gotten to her faster." Gradually, they may come to realize that this was a senseless, horrible accident that robbed them of their daughter and only child. Their dreams for her future died with the phone call from the sheriff. Much has changed in their lives, and they will need to continue to process and adapt to these changes going forward.

The sadness will be with them for the long haul, but their relationship to the loss may change over time, unless one or both parents get stalled in their attempt to move forward. In such an instance, the parent or parents are not able to reconnect with life. Instead, they ruminate about their daughter's death, unable to stop thinking about it, and feeling the sadness as if it happened just yesterday. In other words, their process of adapting has gone off the rails, and they are floundering in a kettle of grief with no visible means of getting out. The loss of their daughter is senseless and horrific, and the grief is still churning after 12 months. These parents and others who are experiencing prolonged grief disorder require professional help to get themselves and their lives back on track.

Please remember that grief experiences may occur with all kinds of losses, and they exist on a continuum. Normative/common grief illustrates what we typically experience when we mourn a loss. There is plenty of room between experiences that are typical and those that may be diagnosed as prolonged grief disorder. We walk our own paths with our grief; our timelines are unique to each one of us. Regardless, getting support is vital in our ability to resume our lives.

Another thing to be aware of is that not all grief is supported in the same way by the larger community. When someone dies, there are usually rituals that follow to support the individual or family that is mourning their loss. Religious and spiritual traditions often guide the process, and neighbors and friends gather round to support those who are grieving with cards, words of encouragement, casseroles, and lending a hand when needed. The grief is recognized, the mourners are supported, and the network is in place to help. Likewise, when your adult child has a debilitating physical illness, friends and neighbors might inquire as to how you are doing and how they can help. They also often share their experiences with their own or a relative's illness, which opens a conversation and provides support. As a result, you feel less isolated and more a part of the larger community.

However, other losses we call living losses, such as losing a job, a relationship, or the dream you had for your adult child who is dealing with a mental illness, are not supported in the same way. Also called nondeath losses, these may be permanent or temporary. Such losses are sometimes referred to as disenfranchised losses (Doka, 1989), where the loss is not recognized or valued and the person experiencing the loss feels they don't have the right to express their grief openly. As a parent you feel intensely the grief of "losing" the adult child you once knew. You try to express this, and your friend says,

"Well at least they're still alive. You can see them every day." Your feelings are tossed aside, and you realize you are not getting the support you need. You are a member of what has been called the "underclass of grievers" (Pine, 1989) who are struggling with a community that doesn't validate the importance of the loss. It is important to keep in mind that such comments from someone indicate their own level of discomfort and their attempt to distance themselves from the loss. The comments reflect the speaker and are not a reflection of you. Let us clarify that the term *disenfranchised loss* can refer to both a death and a nondeath loss experience. The key is the lack of recognition or validation of the loss; with such losses we mourn alone.

Something to keep in mind here as well is that the person who is grieving may not feel entitled to express their grief or to receive support from others. Especially after receiving pushback from those who dismiss or refuse to recognize their loss, the individual or family may try to conceal the loss from others for fear of being condemned or somehow blamed for what occurred. This is often what can occur with a loss through suicide where the stigma is very real and the family members perceive negativity from others, even when it might not actually be there.

Unlike physical losses such as those through death, psychosocial losses, such as having a young adult with a mental illness, are pretty much invisible to the larger community. There is even a tendency to lay the blame at the parent's feet: You must have done something to cause your young adult to develop this condition. Therefore, the support through expressions of sadness or other social or religious rituals is absent. Added to this, is the shame parents often feel about their young adult's situation, the stigma associated with mental illness in general, and sometimes even the parents struggle to accept the loss (MacGregor, 1994).

Although grief is universal, within a family that is sharing a common loss there are as many ways to mourn as there are family members. For that matter, there is no right or wrong way to mourn a loss. It's important to understand that the value you attach to your relationship with the lost object or person is often related to how you will mourn that loss. The more attached you are to the lost person or object, the deeper your sense of grief is going to be.

Additionally, it is important to keep in mind that not all bereavement is visible to the outside world. Some of us are very visible with our grief, whereas others mourn in private. Regardless of how you do it, mourning is the necessary and painful process of doing grief work. It is healthy to do this work, rather than to stay stuck in your grief and let it fester. When we try to bury the grief or bottle up the powerful emotions we feel around our loss, we only set ourselves up for more trouble. All the feelings that get pushed down will resurface with more intensity in other ways, including physical ailments, emotional issues such as anxiety and depression, and problems at work or with our relationships. In other words, these emotions come back to bite us on the butt when we try to keep them at bay.

AVP: ACKNOWLEDGE, VALIDATE, AND PERMIT

We talked with you about the importance of emotion regulation in Chapter 2 and gave you some ways to implement this as you continue your journey with your emerging adult. This skill continues to be essential as you work through loss. "Dr. Becky" offers a skill that she calls a "secret recipe" (Kennedy, 2022, p. 110) for regulating yourself, AVP. The A stands for *acknowledge*, which means just that—identify what you are feeling. "Man, this is rough! My adult child is struggling, and so am I." Or "I'm so scared for my child's safety."

The V stands for *validate*, which means taking your feelings seriously. They are telling you the truth. So you say to yourself, "Wow, trying to handle two jobs, the house and two younger kids, and be there for my adult child who is so depressed is really tough. No wonder I'm feeling overwhelmed right now." Your feelings are not lying to you, you are overwhelmed. Give yourself that validation.

P stands for *permit*: This is about permitting yourself to feel what you feel. Tell yourself, "I'm allowed to feel overwhelmed right now" or "It's okay that I am scared right now." You can even say it out loud if that helps. AVP is a powerful technique for helping you regulate yourself in trying situations such as when you experience a loss. It is also a valuable tool to help you through the process of grief.

👓 MODELS OF GRIEF

Let's look now at some models of grief that we believe are helpful for you to understand more about this experience.

Stage Model

Elizabeth Kubler-Ross is one of the most well-known authors in the field of death and dying. Her famous five stages of death and dying (i.e., denial, anger, bargaining, depression, and acceptance; Kubler-Ross, 2014) mistakenly led folks to believe that there was a stepwise process for moving through their grief. It also set up the expectation that the person who is grieving will, and perhaps should, go through each stage. If you don't experience each stage, you might wonder if you are doing it wrong. David Kessler, who worked with Kubler-Ross toward the end of her life, clarified that these stages were not intended to funnel the grief experience through a stepwise process which ended in resolution. In addition, he added a sixth factor to the mix: finding meaning after a loss, which is an important part of the healing process (D. Kessler, 2019).

Making-Meaning Model

Perhaps more an extension of the stage model from Kubler-Ross than a separate entity, meaning-making nevertheless has arrived front and center in the work of grief. Kessler (2019) and others (Gitterman & Knight, 2019; Neimeyer et al., 2010) have discussed the importance of making some meaning from the loss we have experienced. Please keep in mind that we can and do grieve for losses other than a loss through death, and each of the losses matters because they are important to us. Constructing a new narrative or life story for the person who has lost a loved one, a cherished goal, a place, or even precious time that cannot be recaptured helps that person move beyond the loss and into the next chapter of their life. Losing the hopes and dreams we have for our adult child who is struggling with psychological problems likewise requires such a process. When we create meaning, we find a way to make our loss something we can live with. For some, this means focusing on what was good about the person we lost or what the upside of losing the goal we were striving for is. In doing so we are gaining a new foothold to move ourselves forward with our young adult who is changed, perhaps forever. Rather than staying fixed on how sad we are feeling, a shift in perspective helps us be able to resume our lives, albeit in a different way than we had envisioned.

Some parents find meaning by creating or supporting organizations that are tackling the very issues their young adults are facing. There are many such groups—for example, cancer research and support, addictions support, MADD (Mothers Against Drunk Driving), and NAMI (National Alliance for Mental Illness). These can be powerful aids in the healing process for many of us. We talk more about this in Chapter 10 when we consider the idea of becoming a mental health advocate or doing volunteer work for organizations in the community.

Finding meaning after a loss is a process; it takes time, and there are no shortcuts. Asking ourselves "What can I do with my pain? Where do I go from here?" allows us to begin to imagine that something else is out there. Maybe there is a way to turn the pain into something meaningful and useful for us and perhaps others as well.

Tasks Model

Another way to look at the work of grief is through a task approach, kind of like a to-do list for how to manage. Worden (2008), an internationally known grief expert, gives us a four-task approach to the process of grief and believes all four tasks, although not linear, are essential to working through the pain of loss. Task 1: We must accept that the loss is real. This means recognizing the loss rather than avoiding or denying it. Task 2: We also need to deal with the sadness and pain of the loss. Not all losses carry the same "heaviness" or pain, but it is important for the mourner to engage with the pain they are experiencing. This takes time, and you will have your own way of moving through your loss. Task 3: We must adjust to the world without the person or thing that was lost. Such adjustment happens on three levels: (a) external: how you handle relationships with others, perhaps changes in your daily routine, and so on; (b) internal: how you make meaning of the loss and how you construct a new identity for yourself which takes into account the loss and who you are now; and (c) spiritual: how you incorporate the loss into your worldview (Smith & Delgado, 2020). Task 4: We must emotionally relocate the loss, which means moving it off of center stage in our lives so we can continue on our journey. For example, we will hold the person we've lost in our hearts, but not have them front and center in our thoughts as we go forward. We don't forget them, but they are no longer the central focus of our day.

Again, these tasks are not meant to be linear, but they are each important for the person grieving to work their way through. They will do so based on their own unique makeup, relationship and attachment experiences, and other stressors in their current life circumstances (Worden, 2015). In other words, we each mourn in our own way. You will notice the thread of finding meaning in Worden's approach to grief and mourning. Putting one's assumptive world back on an even keel is another way to look at what the tasks involve.

Dual Process Model

The dual process model of coping with bereavement (Stroebe & Schut, 1999; see Figure 8.3) provides another way to understand what we

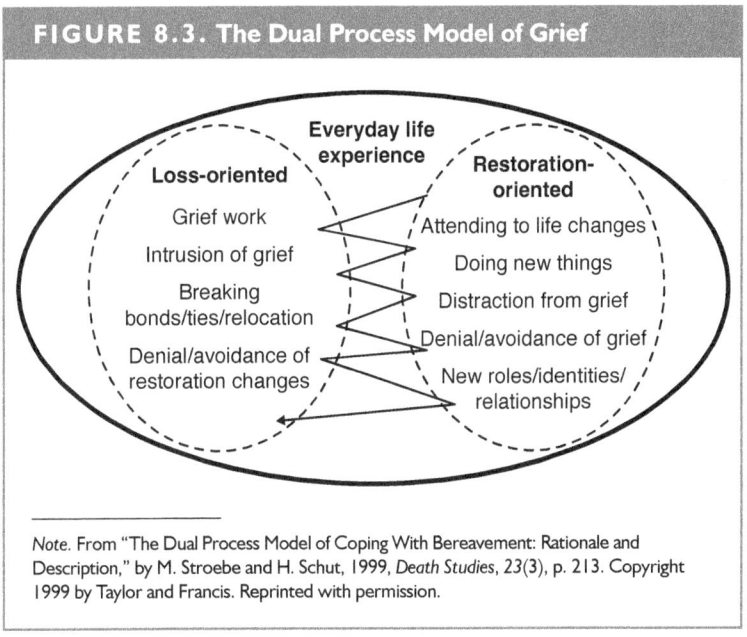

FIGURE 8.3. The Dual Process Model of Grief

Everyday life experience

Loss-oriented
Grief work
Intrusion of grief
Breaking bonds/ties/relocation
Denial/avoidance of restoration changes

Restoration-oriented
Attending to life changes
Doing new things
Distraction from grief
Denial/avoidance of grief
New roles/identities/relationships

Note. From "The Dual Process Model of Coping With Bereavement: Rationale and Description," by M. Stroebe and H. Schut, 1999, *Death Studies, 23*(3), p. 213. Copyright 1999 by Taylor and Francis. Reprinted with permission.

go through when we experience a significant loss. We like this model because the visual provides clarity about the way we go through our days after a loss. This model has three basic components: a loss orientation and a restoration orientation, both of which involve stressors, and an emotional regulation process, known as oscillation.

The loss orientation involves a focus on the loss itself: feeling your sadness and anguish, pushing back against the changes your loss has forced on you. You are caught up in the feelings and struggle to concentrate or begin to move forward. Sometimes this orientation provides a distraction from the tasks ahead as we confront our new circumstances in light of what we have lost. However, we don't want to hang out here to the exclusion of reconnecting with our lives.

The restoration orientation is about revamping your connection to the world that has now changed due to the loss. At a very minimum, this requires you to do something—to shift gears and consider how you move ahead in your life while you mourn your loss. It also involves some effort to move the loss off center stage (denial of the grief you experience) to be able to deal with the changes in your world. The loss doesn't go away; rather you turn your attention away from it for a time to handle your life. Again, just as with the loss orientation being a distraction, the ability to shut out the sadness and grief that it embodies is the very thing we sometimes need to deal with tasks in our changed circumstances.

Oscillation, that zig-zag line between the two, is the "regulator" that requires you to move back and forth between struggling with the loss and focusing on what you need to do now. This regulator pulls you out of the loss and into the future, if you will, and keeps you from getting stuck in either place. You can't sit with your loss all the time, nor can you distract yourself by continually "doing." Moving back and forth between the loss and the restorative functioning through the oscillation process ideally allows you to maintain a balance between the two. It is possible to get overloaded on either side, being consumed by the loss or alternatively in the busyness of trying to move ourselves forward. We need the balance that oscillating between the two sides gives us as we move through our bereavement and into what comes next. Your ability to cultivate emotional awareness and employ emotion regulation are beneficial for you here. In addition, reframing your thinking will further help you to work through whatever loss you have experienced. Exercising these skills also serves to shore up your confidence in your role as wise counsel.

A LONG WINDING ROAD

Let's imagine that the loss you have experienced is a boulder in the road that inhibits your ability to move forward. This can be the case with any type of loss, not just a loss through death. When your young adult has a mental health disorder, the plans you dreamed of their future may no longer exist. Instead, you will need a new plan; first, however, you must recognize the loss of the old one. If you stay focused on the old dream, you will not be able to move forward. Being able to move the old plan off center stage in your life clears the road ahead for a new plan to emerge. This is not the same as denying the loss; rather, it acknowledges what was lost while allowing you to continue your journey. This is an important piece of information for you to absorb.

The Wisdom of Kintsugi

Spanish psychologist Tomas Navarro (2019) talks about the need for emotional strength, which he believes involves three pillars or phases. The first is take a step back. To get a handle on our situation, we first must get some distance from it. Like zooming out on a camera lens, seeing our difficulty from a distance helps us get perspective on it. The second phase, Navarro tells us, is think differently.

He says our thoughts create our reality, so learning to be objective about what we are thinking and how we view the world is important to gaining a clearer picture of what we are dealing with. Without first gaining this new perspective, we are not able to choose an appropriate direction in which to proceed. The last phase, take action, involves mustering our courage and using what we learned from the longer view and a more objective perspective to make and carry out an action plan. Fear can halt us in our tracks here.

"It's scary to think that I can move on from where I am, that my 'broken parts' will hold together and won't push others away from me. I can be present in my life, with all my imperfections, and be okay." When we struggle, when parts of us break, we have the opportunity to grow in ways we would not have imagined before.

Kintsugi, the ancient Japanese art of "golden joinery," is a process that repairs broken pottery in such a way that the breaks are revealed with gold dust (Richman-Abdou, 2022). Rather than cover up the broken spaces, they are in full view as symbols of strength rather than brokenness. Kintsugi can help us practice self-compassion, a concept we discuss in detail in the next chapter. For now, it is important to realize that there is no perfect world, perfect family, or perfect future. And we are not perfect beings. As we learn to embrace our imperfections and understand that we truly can be stronger in the broken places, our ability to be kind and patient with ourselves can only increase our clarity about where we go next.

It's likely there have been many times throughout your journey with your adult child when you felt broken, that your life was in pieces. All you could see were your imperfections. You may feel responsible for many of the challenges your young adult is now facing, such as a failure to launch, symptoms of anxiety and/or depression, unhealthy coping strategies (the dragons), or a serious mental illness. The practice of kintsugi offers yet another strategy to assist in your own self-care.

Given all the ups and downs and even crisis situations you have experienced with your emerging adult in recent years, it's natural to want to hide or disconnect from these memories. Such reminders are often painful and may evoke feelings of guilt and shame. You would like nothing more than to be rid of them, like a scar you want no one to see. Unlike physical scars, emotional scars tend to be invisible, making it easier for you to hide them or keep them to yourself. Unfortunately, keeping such memories to yourself only serves to intensify your pain and reinforce your self-perception of brokenness. Again, as wise counsel this is valuable to know and integrate into a healthier perception of yourself as a person and a parent.

Kintsugi offers a different perspective: Take each of these heart-wrenching memories, imperfections, and shortcomings and view them as proof of your emotional strength and your resilience. Think of all your distressing experiences and memories with your adult child and your perceived inadequacies as pieces of broken pottery. You have a choice: You can either try to discard these pieces (i.e., the past), which is virtually impossible, or you can pick them up and use them to build a new life. You can grow or you can stay stuck in the past. One task of moving forward is to ask yourself to identify what you learned from your past. In this way the past can be helpful as you acknowledge personal growth. Remember, each memory is an important piece of your life journey and therefore deserves to be honored and incorporated as you begin the process of rebuilding. Just as the pottery is rebuilt not as the exact same piece but as something new, so, too, does the process of rebuilding and repairing your own "breaks" result in a new you—someone different, someone stronger.

By applying the concept of kintsugi, we learn to focus on the process of repairing what is broken rather than on the brokenness. It's about looking at your scars differently—not as reflections of brokenness but as reflections of strength. Obviously, this change in perception will take time, but skills learned in previous chapters, such as attending to your inner dialogue and reframing your thoughts, connecting with others, and practicing self-compassion, which you will learn about in Chapter 9, will ease the process and lead to a successful outcome. The goal of kintsugi is to heal. Healing does not mean you will never again experience hardships or challenges, but it does mean you will have the confidence and the necessary tools to cope effectively with whatever demands you may face.

 Taking in the Good

This might be a good place to bring in psychologist Rick Hanson's (2010, 2013) idea of taking in the good. We all know that both good things and bad things happen in our lives. In the natural order of things, our minds have a negativity bias, acting as Velcro for bad stuff, holding on tightly to it, and as Teflon for the good, letting it slip away. To flip this, Hanson offers the skill of taking in the good, that is, focusing on the good things happening around us—the positives of a situation—or pivoting. This is not about stuffing bad feelings down or denying them; they are a part of life. Nor is it about adopting an overly rosy attitude about life. Rather, it is about taking in the good things that happen and good feelings we experience, savoring them, and holding them in our thoughts and our hearts (Hanson & Mendius, 2009). When we do this, we are creating positive memories and a supply of positive thoughts and emotions to counteract the bad ones we inevitably meet. If we look for the good, however, our storehouse will contain more of the positives, thus fortifying our minds and bodies for the journey ahead.

SUMMARY

Loss is a part of living, and we all experience many losses, large and small, during our lives. Our assumptive worlds guide each of us through our daily routines; they operate on autopilot when things are going well. When we experience stress, such as that associated with a loss, our assumptive world may become less stable and "automatic." All losses do not strike with equal force. Although loss is a universal experience, grief is unique to each one of us. The same loss does not affect everyone in the same way. For some of us, even small losses are disturbing, while for others, it takes a significant jolt to shake up our assumptive world. As we engage in the process of mourning our losses, each of us does so in our own way and on our timeline. There is no right or wrong way to mourn, however, it is necessary that we mourn the losses we experience. It is important to remember that not all losses are through death, which is a permanent loss. Other types of loss, such as a physical disability or the development of a mental health disorder in your young adult, can be and often are permanent but do not stem from a death. Models of grief can help us understand what is going on and how we can move through the loss.

Although community support is a vital tool in the mourning process, through religious and spiritual rituals and other forms of coming together to give solace and comfort, not all losses are equally supported. For example, with some living losses like a young adult with a mental health disorder or the loss of a loved one by suicide, support varies widely, ranging from words such as, "Be glad you still have your adult child" to total silence. Whether neighbors and friends don't know what to say or are uncomfortable with the circumstances, they may shy away from encounters with the grieving parents. And the parents themselves may feel they don't have the right to their grief.

Regardless of the loss, many of us can feel broken in its wake. Kintsugi offers us a way to reframe our sense of "brokenness" by accepting and incorporating what feels broken into a stronger and sturdier vision of ourselves going forward. As we look at our imperfections in a different way, we are able to make a decision as to how to move forward in our lives. In the next chapter, our focus is on caring for ourselves through resilience building and the practice of self-compassion. We offer specific strategies to help you tend to your needs so that you are better able to assist your young adult when necessary.

POINTS TO POCKET

- The assumptive world, a set of beliefs we all have about the world, ourselves, and our ability to cope, tends to operate on autopilot until we come face to face with a loss.
- Loss and grief are universal experiences. Each of us mourns the loss and grieves in our own way.
- Losses fall on a continuum and include both nondeath or living losses and death losses. Grief is felt with both nondeath and death losses.
- Models of grief help to explain what we go through as we mourn.
- Community support does not happen equally with all losses, complicating the grief process for the mourner. This is particularly true with a loss by suicide.
- Kintsugi teaches us to embrace our imperfections and gain a new perspective on our losses as opportunities to grow.

CHAPTER 9

TENDING YOUR OWN GARDEN

No one escapes pain, fear, and suffering. Yet from pain can come wisdom, from fear can come courage, from suffering can come strength—if we have the virtue of resilience.
—Eric Greitens, *Resilience*

Up to this point, our focus has been on helping you understand your young adult as they navigate the adulting process in today's tense, chaotic, and unpredictable world, while at the same time keeping yourself on an even keel. As you have seen, emerging adulthood has its own challenges, but many adult children are also facing mental health concerns, which may or may not be accompanied by unhealthy methods of coping. Additionally, in the previous chapter, you read about letting go and the experience of loss, including the loss of your world as you knew it, when your adult child struggles with symptoms of a mental illness. Such a loss is a type of nondeath or living loss, and it is something you can and do mourn. The grief you experience compounds the stress you may already be feeling. To manage this effectively, we recommended earlier that you pivot to and from the roles of caregiver, coach and advanced coach, and wise counsel depending on the situation at hand—that is, the level of functioning and psychological distress in your young adult.

It is likely that until now, you have been focused primarily on meeting everyone else's needs, especially those of your young adult. In other words, you have been tending the gardens of those around you. However, the concepts and strategies described in this chapter can improve your own mental and physical well-being and, in turn, will allow you to be more emotionally available to your young adult, other family members, and friends. Keep in mind, though, you must practice these strategies to reap their benefits.

Self-care and its vital importance to your overall well-being have been mentioned numerous times throughout the book. We already dropped nuggets of self-care suggestions to help you as you process some difficult information. We have identified the basics of self-care as described in the self-care wheel in Chapter 2. We believe self-care is imperative for all parents, especially those whose young adult is in psychological distress.

Our main goal in this chapter is to lead you deeper into the nurturing process of self-care through a discussion of resilience and self-compassion which are integral to taking care of yourself. We break each concept down into skills that you can use in times of distress to feel better about yourself, your decision making, and your overall functioning. Throughout this chapter, we revisit several of the wise counsel skills we presented in Chapter 7 for use with your young adult and weave them into a discussion about taking care of yourself. The foundation of these skills is the ability to empower yourself with new information which involves being open to new ideas. Skills such as reframing thoughts and setting boundaries are essential ingredients for taking care of yourself during times of personal struggle. Furthermore, if these skills communicate a sense of respect for your adult child, why would you not wish to communicate that same message to yourself?

PARENT SELF-CARE

If you find yourself pushing back and saying, "No way! I don't have the time or energy for this!", we hear you! Dealing with the day-to-day challenges of parenting your young adult can leave you feeling physically exhausted and emotionally drained. How on earth can anyone expect you to do even more, let alone take time for yourself? And yet, this is the very point at which self-care can be most essential to your well-being. Rather than viewing self-care as a self-indulgent activity, we see it as a self-nurturing process which allows you to recognize and take care of your own needs. Putting on your oxygen mask first seems totally contrary to what a good parent would do, doesn't it? However, if you aren't breathing, how can you help your adult child?

Don't get us wrong—we love bubble baths and naps! What we want to talk about with you in this chapter, though, moves deeper into the heart of what self-care is and how it can help you. We focus here on *inner work*—the emotions and thoughts that contribute to the exhaustion you are likely experiencing. Many of the ideas you already heard about, such as emotion regulation, cognitive reframing, and radical acceptance, complement and add to what you will learn in this chapter.

Dr. Pooja Lakshmin (2023) talks about the ever-present need for self-care. She views self-care as a verb, not a noun, and she firmly believes it is something we ought to be engaged in on a regular basis, not just when we are struggling. To live a full life and have energy, you must first tend to your own well-being. Self-care is a necessity, not something to think about or maybe do someday. This is important for you regardless of whether you are a mother or a father. Stan, Arturo, and Pete need to employ self-care efforts every bit as much as Claire, Lucia, and Rachel. Taking the time to focus on yourself will not only yield positive results for you personally, but your energy will be freed up to assist others as well.

We strongly believe that self-care is a combination of *resilience-building strategies* and the practice of *self-compassion*. It is important to remember as you continue to read, that we are not adding to the pile of stuff already on your plate. Rather we are asking you to pause and rethink what you are doing and perhaps gain a different perspective on how to include yourself in the mix. After we talk about resilience and self-compassion, we will provide tools specific to self-care for your tote bag.

Parental Resilience

When you hear the word *resilience*, what comes to mind? Maybe being able to bounce back in the face of life stressors? Perhaps the ability to look adversity in the eye and remain standing? If you look up resilience in the dictionary, you will find a variety of definitions, but two components are most always present: the ability to adapt to adversity or tremendous stress and the ability to bounce back. It's important to note that when we say "bounce back," we don't mean a return to the way things were before the adversity struck but rather to reach a point of stability from which to move forward.

Psychological and Behavioral Aspects of Resilience

Researchers have identified both psychological and behavioral components of resilience (Robertson & Cooper, 2013). The psychological aspect allows people to maintain their emotional stability when faced with challenges, both large and small. The behavioral aspect allows people to take action effectively as they face day-to-day stressors. We view the psychological component as a mindset of determination and hope and the behavioral component as the daily steps we take to keep going.

Think of yourself in a boat as a storm approaches the horizon. You see the dark clouds, and you feel the high winds, but rather than panic, you realize you need to adjust your course. You've done this before, and you know you can do it now. By shifting your direction and taking a different course toward the harbor, you head safely away from the approaching storm. Psychologically you maintain your confidence without undue angst and choose to take action to manage the situation rather than becoming its victim. Resilience allows us to hold together when the going gets tough, and when we do tumble, to get back up again.

Let's get into Stan's head as he displays resilience while imagining a possible situation with Anne.

> I've learned a lot about Anne's diagnosis of bipolar disorder by attending the family sessions at the hospital, and it's way more serious than I realized. It scared the hell out of me. You know, I really did not want to go to those sessions, but I feel better now that I know more. It sounds like a lot of people stop taking their medication when they start to feel better. The group facilitator says this can happen when they start into a manic phase. It makes sense that they forget it's the medication that is helping them feel better.
>
> Knowing Anne as I do, I could see her deciding to stop taking her meds once she starts feeling better. They talked a lot in the sessions about relapse, and that also scares the hell out of me. I really don't want to get another call from the police saying that Anne is on her way to the hospital. If it does happen again, though, I feel a bit more prepared. Claire and I have a plan. The first thing we know is Anne could stop her meds. Rather than shaming her for this, we need to look at emergency treatment options that are available to help her.

Stan and Claire understand the cyclical nature of bipolar disorder, and it is this understanding that will help them build resilience. First, they will need to stop, take a breath, and give themselves some time to process their thoughts and feelings. As they move toward understanding that relapse is common, ideally, Claire and Stan will incorporate the possibility of Anne's relapse into their life experience. In doing so, they will be prepared for similar experiences in the future, should they come to pass. Stan and Claire will bounce back but to a new place where they have the tools to cope with the ups and downs of Anne's bipolar illness.

As human beings, we all experience stress, adversity, and pain. When hardship strikes, and it will, resilience offers us both protection and empowerment; it provides us with the resources to cope. The capacity to face hardships with resiliency doesn't mean you eliminate adversity, but it permits you to respond more decisively to whatever your challenges might be. It also involves reaching out to others when you need support. Fortunately, resilience can be developed at any point in time, not just during childhood and adolescence. As a matter of fact, psychologists view resilience as a muscle that can be strengthened over time with practice.

QUALITIES OF PARENTAL RESILIENCE

Many mental health professionals have written about resilience in connection with parenting young children. However, we are focused here on enhancing resilience in the parents whose young adults are experiencing psychological distress. Based on our combined years of clinical experience, we offer you a list of attributes that help fortify resilience in parents of adult children with mental health concerns (Exhibit 9.1). Please remember, these are qualities that can be developed and enhanced over time.

Emotional Savvy. The first quality is what we term *emotional savvy*, the parent's ability to name, accept, and, when necessary, express their

EXHIBIT 9.1. How to Be a Resilient Parent

- Utilize emotional savvy.
- Set boundaries.
- Connect with others.
- Practice cognitive flexibility.

own emotions while being able to listen to and sit with the emotions expressed by their adult child. As we discussed in Chapter 2, the ability to listen with empathy and regulate our emotions is essential. This allows the parent to keep their own emotions in check and their mouth shut while they hear what their adult child has to say. When we talk about regulating our emotions, we are not suggesting that you stuff them down or push them away. All our emotions have value. They help us understand what is going on within us; they send us a signal when something is wrong. Remember, emotion regulation is about clearly identifying your feelings, accepting those feelings, and then making a choice about how to proceed.

Take, for example, a family who owns a farm that has been in the family for decades. The father has always held the expectation that his son would work with him on the farm with the ultimate goal of taking over the farm someday. Then one day his son told him, "I've changed my mind about the farm, Dad. It's more than I can handle. I've been thinking that I'd like to go to college. I've always loved history." Let's listen as Dad talks about the loss he feels:

> I was speechless. My heart started pounding in my chest as I thought about what my son just said. Where did this come from? My son has always, always loved this farm. Our dream of running it together and, one day, him taking over has kept me going through many days when I might have given up. Now he says he doesn't want any part of it. The family business isn't good enough for him. I've devoted my whole life to this and now it's going to end. What would my father and grandfather say?

Dad has a choice to make here. He can go on a rant and tear into his son for turning his back on the family farm. He could guilt-trip his son and try to belittle him into changing his mind. However, he also has the option of demonstrating emotional savvy by first acknowledging his own feelings about the situation and working hard to put these aside for the moment. He then listens intently to his son focusing on his words and his feelings.

> I am very concerned about my son, since this is the first time I've ever heard him express anything remotely like this. He must have been keeping this inside for a long time, and I wonder what it's been doing to him. This isn't the time to be talking about what it's doing to me.

This does not mean that the father can never express his feelings. The option to share is always there, but, right now, he takes time to sit with his feelings for a bit. In doing so, he allows himself time to consider how he can clearly and deliberately communicate with his son.

The father demonstrates emotional savvy by making himself emotionally available to his son. He was fully present with his son as his focus was only on his son. In this case, the father's use of emotional savvy and "holding space" may pave the way for a pivot from wise counsel to compeer down the road. We say more about this pivot in the next chapter.

The father in this scenario was able to acknowledge and tolerate his own negative emotion, something many people find very difficult and challenging to do. The truth is that although negative thoughts and feelings are distressing and uncomfortable, they are also a part of life, and they need to become a part of our life experience. Some people, however, tend to shy away from what is uncomfortable for them.

Have you ever tried to tell someone about something unpleasant you were experiencing, and they immediately came back with "look on the bright side," "it's not that bad," or "cheer up, it will get better?" Such a response may indicate the need to be or appear upbeat and happy all the time. This behavior is called *toxic positivity*, and it means intentionally or unintentionally avoiding, rejecting, or stuffing negative thoughts and feelings. People who engage in toxic positivity believe that painful or negative emotions are bad and should be hidden away. Subsequently, when you tried to talk with them about what you were going through, their toxic positivity immediately shut down the conversation.

It is important to have access to all our emotions, not just the pretty, happy ones. When we are sad or down, it's okay to feel that way, and we don't need people telling us otherwise. Sometimes we even need to experience negative emotions and to think negative thoughts. It is essential to pay attention to and understand what such thoughts and feelings are trying to tell us. By practicing self-compassion, you are in a better position to choose how to proceed when you understand what the negative thoughts and emotions are telling you. For example, if you are feeling overwhelmed and upset, rather than trying to smile, you might need to take action—for example, to reestablish a healthy boundary with those who are encroaching on your space.

Boundaries. The ability to set and maintain *boundaries* is the second quality of parental resilience; this is essential to preserving the parent's sense of self. In Chapter 2, we talked about what it means to have weak, rigid, and healthy boundaries. We expanded this discussion in Chapter 7 to talk about boundaries within a family. Setting healthy boundaries continues to be a part of your journey as a parent. Although all parents benefit from having healthy boundaries with their children, Rachel and Pete may be especially prone to letting their boundaries slip because they are single parents. For many single parents, the effort to be "all things" to their adult children may lead them to neglect their own needs. Later in this chapter, we talk more about the skill of boundary setting, specifically how it relates to your own self-care.

Connection With Others. The third quality of parental resilience is the capacity to develop and maintain *connections with others*—

in other words, being able to reach out and turn to others for support at any time, not only during a crisis. We cannot stress enough the importance of having people in your life whom you can support and be supported by. A good example of the need for connection is with Rachel when her daughter Jessie refused to seek help for her panic attacks and instead chose to share cannabis gummies with her brother.

> I felt such a mix of emotions: I was angry, I was disappointed, but most of all I was scared. I knew I had to talk to someone before I exploded and dumped all of this on my kids. So, I approached my coworker and buddy Jack and asked if he had a couple minutes to talk. We went outside on our lunch break, and as soon as we sat down, I started venting about Jessie. I talked about her anxiety and what dealing with it has been like for me. Boy, what a relief for me to get it all out. Jack just listened, and that was exactly what I needed. Oddly, I felt supported and validated.

Obviously, parenting is not for wimps! It is the hardest job many of us will ever have, and it truly takes a village to be able to care for ourselves as we continue the journey with our young adults.

Cognitive Flexibility. Flexibility reflects the know-how and willingness to adapt to unanticipated changes, both large and small. The fourth quality, *cognitive flexibility* allows you to adapt to changes in your situation; you can sit back and consider various ways of thinking about or looking at the new situation before responding. Reframing your thoughts, discussed in Chapter 5, is an example of cognitive flexibility. We present more information about cognitive flexibility later in this chapter when we look at the benefits of allowing your distressing thoughts simply to be present rather than fighting with them or trying to push them away.

Parents who blame themselves for their adult child's mental health symptoms or problematic behavior likely experience a wide variety of distressing emotions, including guilt, shame, sadness, anxiety, and regret, among others. This is when self-forgiveness can be a vital tool. We define self-forgiveness as a process that involves actively examining the behaviors which you believe resulted in harm to your young adult and understanding that you are not to blame. Ultimately, it is necessary to let go of the negative thoughts and feelings you continue to experience. Self-forgiveness has been shown to improve overall well-being, and it may also assist you in grieving your losses regardless of the nature of those losses.

If you recall the stories of our parents, Claire and Stan, Lucia and Arturo, Rachel, and Pete, the process of self-forgiveness may have had a lot to offer. Claire struggled with the fact that her grandfather carried a diagnosis of bipolar disorder and, rather than talk about it openly, her family's response was to hide it. Claire blamed herself for passing on to Anne the vulnerability to bipolar disorder.

> It's so hard to shake off the memories of my grandfather and how his illness may have contributed to Anne's bipolar diagnosis. In hindsight, I see it more clearly . . . her agitation, the anger toward us. All the signs were there, and still I missed it.

Although Claire wonders if Anne would have been fine had she not inherited her mother's genes, we can see the futility in going down that road. Anne's mental illness was not Claire's fault. Short of not giving birth to Anne at all, there was nothing she could have done to prevent the onset of bipolar disorder. Self-forgiveness is a key tool in helping Claire move on to create a healthier future for herself and her daughter.

With Lucia, similar feelings of guilt and blame emerge.

> When Daniel started going out with Alessandra, I was so sure she wasn't the right girl for him. When she broke up with him,

> I was secretly relieved. I really didn't want to listen to Daniel after the breakup. He was trying to tell me how much pain he was in, and all I felt was relief. How selfish! I should have known better.

Lucia came to believe that in minimizing the loss of Daniel's girlfriend, she may have contributed to his depression. She felt guilty and to some degree responsible for Daniel's symptoms. And yet, Daniel was going through a rough patch that so many young adults will have to experience, and it was not Lucia's fault. To take care of herself, Lucia is better served by a healthy dose of self-forgiveness rather than getting mired in the self-blame game.

Rachel, as well, has something to gain from learning to forgive herself. When Jessie said she was unavailable as a mom due to her hectic work schedule, she also blamed herself and wondered how much of a role she played in Jessie's anxiety.

> I wonder if I put too much on Jessie's shoulders after her dad died. I was so overwhelmed trying to be both parents to Jess and her brother. I had to do it all, there was no one else. I took extra shifts to pay the bills, and left Jessie to babysit Jared. I counted on her help with household chores. She was always so mature and responsible for her age . . . but maybe now as I look back, it was all too much pressure for her. I guess I wasn't around as much as I thought I was.

Once again, beating up on herself keeps Rachel stuck in a negative loop, just like Claire and Lucia.

As is true with Rachel, as a single parent, Pete is also not immune from blaming himself for being overly busy with his work.

> When I was at work, I left Ian alone at home spending more and more time on his computer and less time doing other activities. I couldn't monitor what he was doing every minute of the

day, and he found ways around the controls I did have. I could kick myself now; I should have known better. I'm a teacher and see this all the time at school.

This tendency for parents to blame themselves seems to be deeply embedded. Self-blame in many cases appears to be an automatic response when an adult child engages with one or more of the dragons or develops a mental illness. The preceding cases all illustrate the many ways parents blame themselves when things go wrong. Unfortunately, this tendency is intensified because society often points to the parent and views them as responsible for their young adult's situation.

In a strange way, this blame game that many of us get entangled in is an attempt to control the situation in which we find ourselves. If I take the blame for something, then I have the option to act differently next time and prevent something bad from happening. Likewise, when others point the finger of blame toward us, they have the mistaken belief that they can prevent bad stuff from happening to their own family. In the long run, however, taking the blame or pointing a finger at someone else does nothing to help either the parent or the young adult. This is where self-forgiveness and other tools in your tote bag, like radical acceptance and cognitive reframing, come into play.

Our parents, Claire, Lucia, Rachel, and Pete, could benefit from understanding the essential part that self-forgiveness plays in self-care and how it can lessen the guilt, self-blame, and regret they experience. In addition, they may also be able to let go of their negative thoughts and feelings, thereby making it easier for them to accept what happened and to move on.

Please keep in mind, if you are holding on to the belief that you did something wrong relative to your adult child's mental health status, it's time to let it go. Even if mental illness runs in your family or you regret your parenting style or worry about your life choices (e.g., putting young children in day care, working too many hours), you are not responsible for what has transpired with your young adult. No one is immune from psychological distress or from symptoms of a mental health disorder. Most mental illness is the result of a perfect storm where stress, genetic vulnerability, developmental changes, and other factors come together at a point in time.

Let's look at another aspect of resilience, one that seems to receive less attention. Without a doubt, resilience is about standing up to the challenge, but it is also about something else, and that is learning to bend and flex in the heavy wind rather than remaining rigid. The following Aesop's fable illustrates the point that resilience is as much about choosing to yield and to allow yourself to be flexible in the face of life's demands as it is about resisting and ultimately breaking.

> A Giant Oak stood near a brook in which grew some slender Reeds. When the wind blew, the great Oak stood proudly upright with its hundred arms uplifted to the sky. But the Reeds bowed low in the wind and sang a sad and mournful song.
>
> "You have reason to complain," said the Oak. "The slightest breeze that ruffles the surface of the water makes you bow your heads, while I, the mighty Oak, stand upright and firm before the howling tempest."
>
> "Do not worry about us," replied the Reeds. "The winds do not harm us. We bow before them and so we do not break. You, in all your pride and strength, have so far resisted their blows. But the end is coming."
>
> As the Reeds spoke a great hurricane rushed out of the north. The Oak stood proudly and fought against the storm, while the yielding Reeds bowed low. The wind redoubled in fury, and all at once the great tree fell, torn up by the roots, and lay among the pitying Reeds. (Fables of Aesop, n.d.)

Sometimes it's being flexible, rather than unyielding, that helps us survive and even thrive through challenging and difficult times.

To sum things up, we need both the strength of standing tall and the ability to flex and adapt when necessary to develop resilience.

 ## Parental Self-Compassion

Most of us are familiar with resilience and the concept of self-care. Less well known, and therefore less utilized, is the practice of self-compassion. Self-compassion may be defined as treating yourself with the same level of understanding and kindness that you would provide for a close friend or family member. We want to take a moment here to make a distinction between self-compassion and self-esteem because they are sometimes confused. Self-esteem involves comparison with others and self-evaluation. Self-compassion has no evaluative component. It simply refers to treating ourselves with kindness because we are part of humanity. Kristin Neff (2011), a pioneer in the field of self-compassion research, identifies the three core elements of self-compassion: common humanity (vs. isolation), mindfulness (vs. overidentification—i.e., clinging tightly to negative thoughts/feelings and not living in the present), and self-kindness (vs. self-judgment).

Common humanity, the first element, reminds us that we are human; we are not perfect, and we are not alone. We all feel hurt, we suffer, and we feel personally inadequate at times. These experiences are part of the human condition. Reminding ourselves of our common humanity helps us feel connected to others and this connection can be comforting.

The second element, mindfulness, means being aware of and observing our experiences, thoughts, and emotions from moment to moment, without judgment or resistance (Neff & Germer, 2018). This involves our willingness to acknowledge our uncomfortable feelings without overidentifying with or staying focused on the negative. We talk more in-depth about mindfulness later in this chapter and provide more tools for your tote bag.

Self-kindness, the third and final element of self-compassion, encourages us to treat ourselves kindly. Self-kindness is often mistaken for self-pity. This misunderstanding keeps people from being open to the idea of self-compassion. For example, we often respond automatically with harsh words and self-criticism when something goes wrong. Treating ourselves this way tends to result in feelings of shame: "I am a bad person." This emotion keeps us stuck under a dark cloud. Instead, why not try offering yourself some words of kindness, encouragement, and support—for example, "I made a mistake; this does not mean I am a mistake."

For parents of young adults who are in psychological distress, self-compassion with its three elements is essential for their self-care. As you might expect, self-compassion helps to ease the emotional pain you feel when you experience shock or disappointment, make a mistake, fail at something, or when you just don't like yourself. It helps improve mental and physical well-being, increase motivation, boost connections, facilitate personal responsibility, and decrease symptoms of anxiety and depression (Neff, 2011). In other words, self-compassion builds resilience!

In Chapters 1 and 4, we talked about the role of the brain in the body's reaction to stress—specifically, the fight, flight, or freeze response kicking in when a threat is perceived. What's really interesting to note here is that when the brain picks up on negative self-talk, it reacts the same way as it does to a threat. When our inner dialogue or self-talk constantly berates who we are and what we do, many of those same stress hormones are released, creating what may feel like uncontrollable panic (Neff, 2021). So, when we engage in self-criticism, we end up increasing our stress and hurting ourselves.

Parents, take heart! There is another side to this stress response and its negative impact on our well-being. The practice of self-compassion can also alter our brain chemistry, but in a much different, healthier way. Much like the activation of the stress response system, the practice of self-compassion also results in the release of hormones into the body. These hormones, however, decrease stress and anxiety and promote emotions such as love or warmth. You may have heard of oxytocin. Some people refer to it as the "love hormone." When oxytocin is released in your body, it has a calming effect, slowing your breathing and lowering your heart rate (Neff, 2011). What's not to love?

All the parents in our book have a lot to gain from self-compassion. Claire, Stan, Lucia, Arturo, Rachel, and Pete could continue to douse their brains with stress hormones by engaging in self-blame for their young adults' mental health symptoms. However, there is another choice: They can use self-compassion to combat the stress they experience and enjoy the calming benefits of oxytocin to bring them back to the center. You can enjoy these benefits as well.

Now that you understand the calming effect of self-compassion, we want to introduce you to the other side of self-compassion. Yes, much like resilience, self-compassion has two sides—the "tender" side, as described earlier, and the "fierce" side that originated in Buddhist teachings. Neff (2021) describes this *fierce self-compassion* as "the force that stands up to injustice" (p. 31). Examples of fierce self-compassion include setting and maintaining clear boundaries, verbalizing anger when you feel it, and taking a stand when you feel you have been wronged. Fierce self-compassion helps keep you from being overwhelmed and overrun by another person's actions or attitudes; your boundaries are healthy, and you let the other know where you stand.

Fierce self-compassion can also be practiced when you choose to stand up for others whom you believe are treated unjustly. This could mean advocating for your young adult. Let's use the example of Lucia and Arturo at the hospital following Daniel's suicide attempt. Lucia listened to Arturo yelling at Daniel in the emergency room and telling him he needs to act like a man. This was the last straw for Lucia; she had finally reached her boiling point.

"Enough, Arturo, enough!" she yells at him as she moves between her husband and the hospital bed. "This is our son! He is hurting, and all you do is scream at him." Arturo is dumbfounded; he takes a step back and just stares at her. He has never seen her anger explode before.

"You are a bully, Arturo!" Lucia continues. "You are treating Daniel with no respect. Whenever he does something you don't like, you bully him. Don't you see how he is struggling right now, how he is in pain? He tried to kill himself, and all you can see is how it affects you."

Lucia reaches over and takes her son's hand and states to Arturo, "I won't let you do this to him, do you understand me?"

Arturo doesn't know what to do. He starts to confront Lucia,

"I am the father, and I decide what Daniel needs to be—"

Lucia cuts him off there, and says, "No. *We* are his parents, Arturo. Both of us. We will decide together what he needs, and what we need to do to help him."

Arturo gets angry and starts to storm out. Lucia calls to him, "We need to do this together, Arturo. I can't do it without you."

He pauses at the door, then walks slowly into the hall. Lucia is shaking a bit, she's never talked this way to Arturo before, but it's time. In fact, it's way past time. And it feels pretty darn good, too! She releases a breath she didn't realize she was holding and looks down at her son.

Fierce self-compassion is not always easy to activate, and it can be scary when you have been stuffing down your feelings for a long time rather than recognizing and validating them. Sometimes it takes an emotionally charged situation to get us going. Lucia had been the silent one for so long, enduring her husband's rants about their son and not speaking up. Seeing Daniel lying in the bed in the

ER, she could not be silent anymore. Like a mother bear protecting her cub, Lucia took action and stood up for her son. In doing so, Lucia also took care of herself. Fierce self-compassion can be an active part of self-care.

Neff (2021) refers to these concepts, tender and fierce, as the yin and yang of self-compassion. Yin and yang are two interdependent concepts of Chinese philosophy representing opposites, and one cannot exist without the other. A frequently cited example of yin–yang is night and day; you can't have day without night and vice versa. The same is true of the tender and the fierce sides of self-compassion: they are opposites that work best in harmony. Ultimately, the goal of self-compassion is to alleviate our suffering; sometimes we speak comforting words to ourselves and other times we get angry and demand respect for us and for others. Self-compassion, when practiced in balance, can contribute significantly to our overall mental and physical well-being.

PARENTAL SELF-CARE IN ACTION

Believe it or not, you already have the skills to practice self-compassion. You have offered compassion to friends and family for years. Your challenge now is to apply these same skills to yourself. This may seem like a foreign concept because our culture tends to socialize us to be hard on ourselves rather than compassionate. For so many of us, our immediate response when something goes wrong is to beat ourselves up, rather than to offer ourselves kindness and understanding. Unlike how we would respond to a friend, we seem to view ourselves as undeserving of compassion. We may even hold on to the faulty belief that the harder we are on ourselves, the more motivated we will be, and ultimately, the happier and more successful. Interestingly, research has shown this to be untrue (Craig et al., 2020; Powers et al., 2007; Wakelin et al., 2022). In fact, it's just the opposite. Self-compassion leads to increased overall wellness; in other words, the more compassion or kindness you give to yourself, the more emotionally available you will be to others. Through the practice of self-compassion, you can become the best possible you!

Mindfulness: An Act of Parental Self-Care

As mentioned earlier, mindfulness refers to being fully aware of our here-and-now experience—our thoughts and feelings—and accepting it without imposing judgment. In other words, we are willing to acknowledge and be with whatever uncomfortable feelings we may have. We've noted that mindfulness is one of the components of self-compassion. Let's take a moment and learn what it feels like to be in the here and now by practicing the following exercise.

Find a small stone that you find especially attractive. Then try the following exercise:

- Start by carefully examining your stone. Notice the colors, the angles, and the way the light plays on the surface of your stone. Allow yourself to enjoy the sight of the stone.
- Now explore the stone with your sense of touch. Is it smooth or rough? What is the temperature?
- Let yourself become absorbed in your stone, pouring yourself into the experience of handling this beautiful stone.
- Allow yourself to experience your stone with all your senses, appreciating its uniqueness.
- Notice that when you are focused on your stone, with appreciation, there is little room for regret or worry, for the past or the future. You are "at home" in the present moment. (Neff & Germer, 2018, p. 48)

This exercise helps to sensitize us to the difficulties of staying in the present moment. We may begin to realize how powerful a tool mindfulness can be, and just how often our thoughts slide into the past or jump ahead to the future. We are able to see how rarely our thoughts are focused on the present moment.

Once we become aware of our distressing thoughts and feelings, we can choose to see them as just thoughts and associated emotions— not necessarily an objective reflection of reality. It is the ability to sit with our pain that allows it to dissipate. We need to turn toward our pain before we can respond to it with compassion. Mindfulness provides us with the time and space to respond in a compassionate way.

In Chapter 5, we talked about the power we give our self-defeating thoughts. Before we know it, we are tangled up in these thoughts and believe them to be true. In his book *Don't Believe Everything You Think*, Joseph Nguyen (2022) describes a connection between our suffering and the credibility we give our thoughts. He explains that thoughts just pop into our heads, and we have no control over that. However, where we get into trouble is when we spend too much time dwelling on our thoughts and ultimately giving them power over how we feel and what we do. This unfortunately can lead us into a downward spiral of sadness, anxiety, regret, anger, and so on, due to the strong connection between our thoughts and feelings. We do, however, have control over how we choose to respond to our thoughts. The following folktale clearly captures this choice:

> An old Cherokee chief was teaching his grandson about life. "A fight is going on inside me," he told the young boy, "A terrible fight between two wolves." "One is evil, full of anger, sorrow, regret, greed, self-pity, and false pride. The other is good, full of joy, peace, love, humility, kindness, and faith." "This same fight is going on inside of you, grandson . . . and inside of every other person on this earth." The grandson ponders this for a moment and then asks, "Grandfather, which wolf will win?" The old man smiled and simply said, "The One You Feed." (The Academy for Professional Excellence, 2015)

We almost always have a choice; we can either give power to our negative, self-defeating thoughts or we can give power to our positive, optimistic thoughts.

The practice of mindfulness allows us time to reflect on our thoughts and to decide how we want to respond to them. When practicing mindfulness, you are aware of your negative thoughts, but you choose not to judge the thoughts or yourself for having the thoughts. You sit back and observe them. In so doing, you are neither giving power to your thoughts nor are you trying to avoid or push the thoughts away. You simply allow them to be present. This gives you time to choose how you want to respond. Remember you can do nothing to change the past, nor do you have control over the future, but you can do something in the present moment.

Self-compassion is needed when we are suffering and in pain. Have compassion for your pain. Don't try to ignore it as so many people do. Pain has the power of persistence; the more you try to avoid it, the stronger it becomes. Be kind to yourself just as you would be to a close friend. Remember you are not alone. We are all in this big pot of humanity together. Reach out to others who will be with you while you are hurting.

Just as mindfulness can be helpful in managing negative emotions, it also affords you the opportunity to get the most out of all your experiences. It helps you stay focused in the present, and it reduces distractions. Mindfulness makes it possible for you to recognize pleasurable as well as negative experiences. You often have the option to repeat the enjoyable experiences at a future time. We must remember that where there is negative, there is also positive; they coexist, and we have the power to determine where we choose to focus.

Reframe Your Thoughts: An Act of Parental Self-Care

In Chapter 5, we encouraged you to change your mindset by challenging negative thoughts and replacing them with more positive, rational thoughts. We pointed to the connection between negative self-talk and how we respond poorly to others or undermine ourselves. The ability to reframe your thoughts and move beyond negative self-talk is an important part of self-compassion. Let's now look at some useful ideas from acceptance and commitment therapy (ACT; Harris, 2009) a psychological intervention introduced in Chapter 5, that advocates a focus on the here and now to adapt to the situation at hand and make a decision in line with one's goals and values. This approach teaches us how to stop avoiding or struggling with uncomfortable thoughts and emotions. It also encourages us to notice, be open to, and to accept negative emotions. When we accept rather than resist or fight such emotions, any anxiety or stress we are experiencing decreases. The calmer we feel, the more capable we are of facing whatever situation awaits us. When we are relaxed and in control of our emotions, we can commit to a course of action that aligns with our personal values and goals.

ACT uniquely offers metaphors to help readers relate to its concepts, making it easier to apply them to their own lives. For the purposes of this book, we have selected two examples of metaphors that reflect what happens when we resist rather than accept our thoughts and feelings.

Consider the first example: a ball in a pool.

 BALL IN A POOL

> What if what you're doing with these thoughts, memories, and feelings is like fighting with a ball in a pool? You don't like these things. You don't want them, and you want them out of your life. So you try to push the ball under the water and out of your consciousness. However, the ball keeps popping back up to the surface, so you have to keep pushing it down or holding it under the water. Struggling with the ball in this way keeps it close to you, and it's tiring and futile. If you were to let go of the ball, it would pop up and float on the surface near you and you

probably wouldn't like it. But if you let it float there for a while without grabbing it, it could eventually drift away to the other side of the pool. And even if it didn't, at least you'd be able to use your arms and enjoy your swim, rather than spending your time fighting. (Stoddard & Afari, 2014, p. 39)

The truth is the more we struggle with and resist uncomfortable thoughts and feelings, the more intense and relentless they become. Let's assume each ball represents a negative thought you may have experienced as the parent of a young adult with mental health concerns. Examples of such thoughts could be the following: "You did this, you screwed up your kid," "It's all your fault," or "How could you not have seen this coming?" Does any of this sound familiar to you? The more we get hooked into the thoughts, the more and more entrenched in our brains they become, which then leads to rigid thinking patterns. Rigid thinking often results in poor decision-making and a very negative view of self.

It would not be surprising if this metaphor rang true for you. People instinctively seem either to push away uncomfortable thoughts or try to deny their existence. The truth is, the more we struggle with and resist uncomfortable thoughts and feelings, the more intense and relentless they become. The thoughts become firmly ingrained in our brains and our thinking becomes very rigid, a sign of poor mental health. Rigid thinking interferes with our ability to think clearly, identify viable solutions to problems, and make sound decisions.

This next example offers a different approach to managing distressing thoughts and feelings.

Floating Leaves on a Moving Stream

Imagine sitting by a stream on a warm, sunny day, watching the leaves float by. Now become conscious of your thoughts. Each time a thought pops into your head, imagine that it's written on one of those leaves. If you think in words, put them on the leaf as words. If you think in images, put them on the leaf as images. The goal is to stay beside the stream and allow the leaves to keep floating by. Don't try to make the stream go faster or slower. Don't try to change what shows up on the leaves in any way. If the leaves disappear, if you mentally go somewhere else, or if you find that you're in the stream or on a leaf, just stop and notice that this has happened. File that knowledge away and then once again return to the stream. Watch a thought come into your mind, place it on a leaf, and let the leaf float downstream. Continue for the next few moments, just watching your thoughts float by. (Stoddard & Afari, 2014, p. 38)

As you read this metaphor, were you able to imagine your thoughts on a leaf floating peacefully down the stream and away from you? Could you feel the contrast between pushing your thoughts down and allowing them to be there until they passed? Simply observing your thoughts, rather than getting into a fight with them, gives you the time and space to think clearly about how you choose to proceed. Before we move on to a discussion of mindfulness, let's take a moment to revisit the wise counsel skill of setting and maintaining boundaries.

Setting Healthy Boundaries: An Act of Parental Self-Care

Boundary setting was discussed in Chapter 7 specifically as it relates to types of boundaries and the impact each type can have on the functioning of the family unit. Here we are focusing on the ability to set boundaries as an integral part of self-care although establishing them can feel challenging at times. Parents, especially moms, become accustomed to putting their needs aside and prioritizing the needs of others, particularly their children. Although it can be rewarding to attend to the needs of others, it can result in a loss of self. For example, imagine you are getting ready to go to the gym to work out when your adult child shows up at your house and says, "Hey mom, I had this afternoon off and decided to come and hang out with you." You respond saying, "I'm so glad to see you, but I was just on my way out. I'm headed to the gym to work out." Your young adult says, "But mom, I don't know when I'll have another afternoon off." You say, "I realize that, but I had an extremely stressful week, and my workout is what keeps me in a good place. I'm sorry, but I really need this workout. Why don't we look at our schedules and find another time?"

Lakshmin (2023) sees boundary setting as the foundation of self-care and, therefore, as imperative. It's so easy to assume friends, family, and coworkers will know when you've reached your limit, and you hold the unspoken expectation that they will jump in and help. Often, this doesn't happen, and you begin to feel angry and resentful. One viable solution is for you to set boundaries for yourself; for example, make your limits known, agree to get back to them later. Setting boundaries is effective in helping you regain or maintain your sense of self.

> As a single dad, Pete has always had an ongoing struggle with setting boundaries with his son. He does well at work with students and coworkers but has a hard time with Ian. On the one hand, he knows that time for himself and his responsibilities is important; on the other hand, he is the main support for Ian and has a hard time putting his own priorities first.
>
> "I know in my head that boundaries help me to maintain my sanity as a single dad, but Ian tugs at my heartstrings, and it's hard to say no without feeling guilty. I'm getting better at it, but I still need a lot of work on this!"

Here are three basic boundary-setting strategies to keep in mind. First, it is essential as a parent that you identify your wants and needs and that you communicate them; let people know where you stand.

Second, live according to your values. Don't feel the need to compromise them for the sake of others. And third and, maybe most important, say no when you want to without assuming guilt. Saying no can sometimes be the hardest thing to do, especially when you have given in in the past. Setting healthy boundaries is good for your mental health, and it reduces stress!

A caveat to remember when setting healthy boundaries: They are flexible and allow you to adapt them to the needs of the situation. For example, if Rachel, in the situation above, sensed that Jessie was really struggling with her anxiety, she may choose to change her plans and respond more immediately to her daughter's request. When your boundaries are healthy, you can make decisions about when and how to alter the plan based on what is right in front of you. Unlike weak boundaries, where you cave in to the needs of everyone, or rigid boundaries, where you won't budge, healthy ones put you in the driver's seat and allow you to pivot as the situation changes.

SUMMARY

We hope what you learned in this chapter has both expanded your definition of self-care (i.e., a combination of resilience-building skills and self-compassion) and enhanced your desire to practice it. We strongly believe the skills presented here, when employed regularly, can reduce your feelings of anxiety, sadness, and distress, while giving you some sense of control over your life. Self-care is imperative for parents of young adults with or without a mental health disorder who are trying to find their way through emerging adulthood in today's unpredictable and often topsy-turvy society. Parental resilience refers to the ability either to "stand tall against" or to "flex with" life's ever-changing circumstances. In our experience, parental resilience consists of the following four key qualities: emotional savvy, boundary setting, connection with others, and cognitive flexibility. These qualities can be developed or improved at any point in life, and doing so strengthens resilience. Self-forgiveness is an option for those parents who continue to blame themselves for their young adult's mental health symptoms or psychological distress. The process of self-forgiveness allows parents to let go of their guilt and self-blame, thereby improving their mental well-being. Self-compassion is a foundation of self-care; it refers to treating yourself with kindness and understanding, just as you would a friend. It's essential to understand that there are two sides to self-compassion: the tender side and the fierce side. They are most effective when practiced in balance with one another. Toward the end of the chapter, we offered specific self-care strategies—mindfulness, cognitive flexibility, and boundary setting—to add to your tote bag.

In the next chapter, we summarize the main themes and highlights of your journey throughout our book. We present the final pivot point, that of a compeer or a "trusted companion." We stress the aspirational nature of this role as well as the importance of knowing when to pivot to a previous role. As we mentioned earlier, your decision to pivot is based on your young adult's degree of psychological distress and level of functioning. Specific tools to assist you in developing the mindset and skills of a compeer will be provided. Finally, we will have one last visit with Claire, Stan, Lucia, Arturo, Rachel, and Pete and bring their stories to a close.

POINTS TO POCKET

- Adversity is a given, but resilience is learned.
- Take time to assess each situation and then decide. Do I need to stand strong, or do I need to flex?
- Self-care is not a to-do list; it is a way of life.
- Self-compassion means treating yourself as you might a friend.

- Practice both sides of self-compassion—the tender and the fierce. Treat yourself with kindness and stand up for what you believe.
- Stay in the here and now; allow your thoughts to be there and then decide how to respond to them; say no when you know it's the right answer.

CHAPTER 10

THE COMPEER STATE OF MIND

There is a crack in everything, that's how the light gets in.
—Leonard Cohen, *Anthem*

"Some days are diamonds, some days are stones. Sometimes the hard times won't leave me alone" (Denver, 1981). So sings John Denver with words that may feel quite familiar to you as the parent of an emerging adult. No matter what your personal circumstances are, the world we live in is chaotic and unpredictable. Depression, anxiety, and other forms of psychological distress in emerging adults continue to steadily rise even after the COVID pandemic has passed. Your job description during the stage of emerging adulthood has become more complex and multifaceted. It's been quite a ride so far, hasn't it, Mom and Dad? Kudos to you for hanging in there!

As you begin this final chapter, you may be feeling somewhat overwhelmed. Perhaps you are asking, "Now, when was I supposed to pivot? And how do I validate my young adult without interfering? How can I offer help without enabling them?" If these questions are buzzing around in your head, you are in good company. In this chapter, we return to our parent pivoting wheel and a new pivot for parents: from wise counsel to compeer. In our parenting model, the word *compeer* refers to the combination of qualities of a "companion" and "peer." In compeer mode, you build on the skills acquired from previous pivots. We offer some new skills and additional ways to care for yourself.

We return one last time to our parents—Stan and Claire, Arturo and Lucia, Rachel, and Pete—and their emerging adults who are on the brink of full-fledged adulthood. For both parents and their adult children, life has been disrupted to varying degrees, and hence their futures are uncertain. The assumptive worlds of these parents have been rocked to varying degrees; in some cases, they have been shattered. As you learned in Chapter 8, these once taken-for-granted belief systems sometimes require a reset as the parents struggle to come to terms with their new normal. You will hear in our parents' stories some degree of uncertainty about what the future may hold for them and their emerging adults.

Are you ready? Pick up your tote bag, put on your spectacles, and let's venture forward into a compeer state of mind.

👓 PIVOT TO COMPEER

To better understand the compeer role, take a moment to consider how you would describe a trusted companion. Qualities such as being supportive, empathetic, nonjudgemental, fun to be around, for example, might come to mind. As a parent in the compeer mode, you embody these attributes as well as the ability to care about and respect your young adult without feeling the need to take care of them. In the compeer role, you take your foot off the gas pedal, at least for a while, and allow yourself to coast, knowing that your adult child is doing well on their own. You trust that they can be responsible for themselves, just as you take responsibility for yourself and your actions. Just as a trusted companion might seek out your advice on occasion, so, too, might your young adult do the same. Likewise, you might ask for their input on an issue with which they are more savvy. How many of us have welcomed our young adult's superior expertise on matters of technology, for example?

As we have demonstrated, maintaining healthy personal and family boundaries, employing emotion regulation, and reframing unhelpful thoughts are essential for parents of young adults. In the previous chapter, we underscored the need to expand the conventional definition of self-care beyond simply a list of wellness activities by using the tool of self-compassion. This means showing yourself the same kindness that you would show to others, including your emerging adult. Self-compassion is an essential tool to carry with you into the compeer role.

Now that we have given you an idea of what the compeer role looks like, we must acknowledge that when your adult child is experiencing a serious mental health issue, the pivot to compeer may not be feasible and may even be ill advised. Although compeer is something we might all aspire to, the very real needs of our adult children may have us pivoting to a different role. It is imperative that you meet them where they are in their psychological distress and level of functioning and adapt your pivots accordingly.

We know that relapse can and often does happen with serious mental illness and that you will likely need to pivot to caretaker, coach, or advanced coach again. There is no way to predict the course of a serious mental health disorder in young adults. For some of them, the need for assistance or mentoring from someone—not necessarily parents—may continue throughout their lives. Remember in Chapter 8 we emphasized the importance of "taking in the good" (Hanson, 2010). Holding on to the positives is a way to increase the strength and resilience you need to continue the journey.

Some parents may have few opportunities to be a compeer with their adult children; that's not a failure on anyone's part. It is possible to operate in compeer mode for a period of time, and then, if something unexpected happens, you pivot to one of the other roles. You may return to each of the earlier ones for a time and eventually reach compeer again. As you know by now, the pivots we describe are fluid rather than stationary, and as a parent, you will move in and out of them based on the situation with your adult child. Remember to keep that pivoting wheel well greased! Regardless of the role or point on the pivoting wheel, give yourself and your emerging adult permission to be what Ann Douglas (2023) termed "gloriously imperfect."

 SKILLS FOR THE COMPEER STATE OF MIND

As you learned from the previous pivots, there are skills associated with each of the parenting roles. We turn now to the compeer mindset and remind you that the new skills we present here build on all you have learned so far in this book. So polish up those skills from the other roles and step into the compeer state of mind. Exhibit 10.1 offers a list of skills essential for the compeer to acquire. We hope these will help you improve your relationship with yourself and others, as well as with your young adult.

Welcome Contact and Maintain Healthy Boundaries

Connections between parent and adult child naturally ebb and flow as you pursue your own paths. If you live in close proximity to them, this may help you keep a close link with them. These days,

---

EXHIBIT 10.1. How To Be a Compeer for Your Adult Child

- Welcome contact and maintain boundaries.
- Develop a curious mind.
- Own your stuff.
- Enhance the positive.
- Find meaning through action and connection.

---

however, you don't need to live nearby to stay in touch. You have several options available to you thanks to technology. Video chats, email, texting, and so on allow you to connect with your young adult regardless of the distance. And, as with any convenience, there is good news and bad news when it comes to using such tools. While they help you stay in touch with your emerging adult, with email and texting, the full message doesn't always come through, and misunderstandings may occur in both directions. Be mindful of the importance of clear deliberate communication in texts and emails. In these times of "textese" and cutesy emojis, your intended message may not be perceived accurately. Such links through technology are also less satisfying than face-to-face conversations, although sometimes they are the best you can do given the circumstances.

When you live close to your young adult, you may be tempted to drop in unannounced for a visit, which can often seem to them as an invasion of their space. In the same way, you can overdo the use of technology, calling, texting or attempting to reach them on a video link more often than is reasonable. Wanting to connect with your young adult is healthy, but insisting on it daily, even multiple times a day, can lead to trouble.

As a compeer, you understand the importance of maintaining healthy boundaries in relationships. This is crucial in your relationship with your young adult. As a parent you may want to say something about their lifestyle, choice of partner, or work situation. However, in a compeer state of mind, you understand that they are responsible for their choices, not you. You refrain from giving advice or making judgmental statements because you trust their ability to handle themselves and make good decisions. Closeness and respect are enhanced when you are able to close your mouth and open your mind. What we are talking about here is the opposite of making an unannounced visit to your young adult, offering advice they didn't request, or assuming a level of contact that they haven't agreed to.

Imagine that you haven't seen your good friend in over a month. You invite them to lunch and are looking forward to an afternoon together. When they arrive, they inform you that they have about 45 minutes before they will have to leave to pick up a friend at the airport. Your immediate internal reaction is disappointment and sadness, with a sprinkling of anger. However, although human emotion may bubble up, you respond by expressing mild disappointment but, at the same time, enjoying the time that you have together.

Now, imagine the same scenario. This time you are having lunch with your adult child. Talk about an exercise in self-restraint, Mom and Dad! In a compeer state of mind, you enjoy every minute of the lunch knowing the time is limited.

As you know, the balance of power changed as your young adult began their journey through this emerging adult phase of their life. In some cultures, adult children are expected to defer to what is good for the family and to be subservient to the needs of their elders. In our Western society, this journey looks different: You are transitioning from a parent–child relationship to a more adult–adult relationship. This means that either one of you can initiate and even finance an outing or recreational activity with the other (going to a ballgame, catching a movie, having lunch at a new restaurant in town). Remember, it is the quality of time, rather than the actual amount of time, that counts.

Develop a Curious Mind

When we have a curious mind, we are open to new and at times unexpected or even shocking ideas, opinions, and information that we may not have been exposed to or even entertained before. Curiosity is a way of showing interest in the new and novel, which leads us to try to understand what is unfamiliar rather than reject it out of hand. We might, for example, do a little objective research on our own to understand what is unfamiliar to us. Curiosity also assists us in understanding the feelings and thoughts of another person. We gain information by listening and asking a series of questions with the end goal of a conversation.

When your young adult makes a life choice, such as taking a job in Oregon when they've never been out of Nebraska before, you may have a shock moment! Hold on, Mom or Dad! We know your apprehension is rising. Rather than reacting with judgment, take a breath and consider: What is it about this job that would draw them away from the familiar and into such unknown territory? In other words, get curious, learn more, and give them space to tell you about their choice. Your ability in this moment, once again, to shut your mouth and open your mind, will keep you in the compeer mindset. And your young adult is more likely to talk about their decision rather than hang up on you or storm out the door. You might also consider contacting your old college roommate, who now lives in Oregon, and asking what it's like to live there. If you make your default mode curious, not reactive, you convey to your emerging adult that you respect and trust their decisions. You also increase the chances that this won't be the last conversation you have about the issue.

Own Your Stuff

Having a curious mind helps us gain an understanding of the world around us, and this includes our adult children and the decisions they make. As we open our minds to new ideas as well as old, we may come face to face with some of our own vulnerabilities that we've tried to keep at bay. Rather than ignoring them any longer, it is useful to "own our stuff" and understand how it may have impacted our parenting. An honest effort to confront these little "imperfections" in ourselves goes a long way to taking away their power over us. It also diminishes the power they might have in our relationships with others.

Once we take an honest look at ourselves and begin to acknowledge and deal with our shortcomings, we are in a better place to respond nondefensively when others point them out. For example, imagine you are having a phone conversation with your young adult but finding yourself distracted by a pressing problem at work. They sense your distraction and call you on it, yelling into the phone that you never listen. You always let work interfere when they are talking to you. In your head, you automatically start formulating your defense, but they hang up.

You ask yourself, is this true? Have I often been distracted by my work concerns? This pause before responding allows you to ask the honest question of yourself. The answer is an uncomfortable but very clear yes. Now you have the opportunity to respond nondefensively and be able to listen without feeling the need to correct them. You call your adult child back and apologize for your behavior, telling them it's something you will work on.

Sometimes it can be a difficult pill to swallow having to admit to yourself, and your adult child, your own vulnerability and mistakes. However, when you do, it affords the opportunity to strengthen the relationship. You own your stuff without needing to justify your behavior, and by doing this, you allow for a different outcome. Nondefensive listening and responding opens up the pathways of communication and allows both parties to be heard. Again, remember that you as a parent are "gloriously imperfect" (Douglas, 2023). And that's okay, Mom and Dad!

Enhance the Positive

Take a deep breath and imagine you are sitting to with your first cup of rich coffee in the morning, or you just walked into the local bakery and were immediately greeted by the aroma of chocolate chip cookies right out of the oven. Ummm . . . is your mouth watering? These are pleasant experiences that you may want to hold on to. Just as you might savor these rich aromas, so too can you learn to savor moments of joy and happiness when they happen with your young adult.

In previous chapters we talked about the importance of regulating negative emotions. It is equally important to embrace and enhance our positive emotions (joy, contentment, happiness, etc.). Let's take a look now at the contributions of positive psychology, a specialty that promotes the study of personal strengths and qualities that help us to flourish (Peterson & Seligman, 2004; Seligman, 2012; Seligman et al., 2005).

One such quality that has significant benefits is a sense of humor. Cultivating and maintaining a sense of humor allows us to see the funny—and at times absurd—side of life, and can help prevent us from taking ourselves too seriously at times. Positive psychologists consider humor to be a "character strength," or a trait that enables us to flourish. Humor and shared laughter bind and connect us to one another and are considered a form of play (Martin & Ford, 2018). Humor helps us to cope with stressful or awkward situations by helping us shift our perspective or frame of mind. Healthy humor not only enhances and prolongs positive emotions like joy and contentment, it also fosters resilience and improves our physical well-being by slowing our heart rate, lowering blood pressure and reducing stress. In addition, humor can help us get out of a negative mindset and shift our perspective, perhaps allowing us to focus more on the positives around us. Who knew that a good belly laugh could be such a gift?

We will issue a caveat about humor: Healthy humor allows us to laugh with another person, not at them. We can also laugh at ourselves. What we don't want to do is use humor to demean or denigrate another person, or ourselves. So whether we are laughing with others or at ourselves, the key is to do it kindly and in good fun. When we make light of our own behaviors or goof-ups, we can enhance our connection with others ("See, I can make mistakes, too!") rather than putting others off ("I would never do something stupid like that"). We show our humanity through our ability to laugh at ourselves. Humor is not a weapon with which to attack our enemies; rather, it is a tool to lighten the mood, the journey, and the atmosphere in the room. Humor is our ally as we move through life, and if we use it wisely, there will be more joy and laughter coming our way.

So how do we bring more humor and therefore more joy into our lives? We're confident you already have some skill in this area. Here are a couple more things you might do. First of all, hang around funny people—that is, people who employ healthy humor, who you can laugh with, and who will laugh with, not at, you. Watch funny movies or TV programs you enjoy. Keep funny greeting cards or sayings, maybe post them on your refrigerator to see as you pass through the kitchen each day. Turn off the news and turn to a funny book for a change of mood and mindset. Once you get the humor juices flowing, you will begin to see the funny elements in everyday life right alongside the challenges. If you create space for laughter and joy in your life, you won't have to go looking for it; it will come to you. Try to have at least one good belly laugh a day. You will be amazed at what it can do for you!

There is a theory in positive psychology called "broaden-and-build" developed by Barbara Fredrickson (1998, 2013) which says that when we feel positive emotions such as we might after completing a huge home improvement project, we may be momentarily filled with ideas of other projects to tackle, or ways to celebrate what we've accomplished. Our positive feelings lead to an expansion or broadening of our thoughts, which become linked to actions. This means that we can think more creatively and act in ways that enhance our well-being. Over time, the joy we experience leads to more and more joy.

Let's contrast this expansive, creative activity with what happens when we experience negative emotions, such as fear and anxiety. These are accompanied by a narrowing of immediate thoughts and limited range of actions in the interest of self-protection. When the driver ahead of you appears to be drifting into someone else's lane, your fear narrows your thinking, you are in tunnel-vision mode, and your thoughts constrict to survival: "He's going to kill us or somebody else." You quickly jump into action and change lanes or take the next exit to literally distance yourself from the suspicious driver. Your response is another example of the flight, fight, or freeze response described in Chapter 1.

Practitioners of positive psychology have developed some creative ways to enhance pleasant feelings. One way to do this is to keep a gratitude journal where you list things, experiences, people who give you joy. You can also write a letter of gratitude to someone you want to thank or engage in simple acts of kindness. Or try the gratitude exercise in Exhibit 10.2.

EXHIBIT 10.2. Gratitude Exercise

Find a comfortable seat and close your eyes. Imagine you have a basket in front of you that you are going to fill with people and things you enjoy, experiences you love, thoughts that bring you happiness. Get a picture in your mind of these positive influences and begin putting them in the basket one by one. Keep putting these things in your basket, and as it starts to overflow, imagine a larger basket. As you continue to focus on this positivity, allow yourself to really feel and savor the joy you are experiencing. Breathe in the happiness and hold it close.

Note. Data from LaFreniere (2023).

Savoring is another technique that helps us increase our positive feelings. Intellectually, we can define savoring as the capacity to attend to, relish, and enhance positive emotions associated with positive events (Bryant & Smith, 2015; Bryant & Veroff, 2007). In practical terms, savoring enhances our mood: We feel happy, which can help promote resilience and also physical and psychological health.

So how do you savor a moment with your young adult? Let's consider the following example. You are out at the bookstore in town, and they walk through the door. This is an unexpected happy surprise. They come up to you and give you a hug. You proceed to wander up and down the aisles talking about the books you've read and the ones you want to buy. You are enjoying this unexpected delight of spending some quality time together. They leave after 20 minutes to continue with their day, and as you pay for your books and head out, you are filled with happiness for this golden moment. You look forward to more such moments in the future. At dinner, you tell your partner about this happy surprise with your young adult. Before crawling into bed, you note the unexpected encounter in your gratitude journal. Later in the week, as you prepare for a difficult meeting at work, you return to the feeling of happiness you had with your young adult. It helps you calm yourself before you enter the meeting room.

We can develop and increase our ability to savor by using our thoughts and behaviors. For example, thinking about how much we enjoyed an experience and holding on to the feelings it brings up in us can help to retain the moment. Also, smiling, reaching out to thank someone, or sharing the pleasurable experience with another person can help to reinforce the positive vibes we feel. Before we can savor a moment, we have to recognize that something good has occurred and then reinforce it with our thoughts or actions to increase the likelihood it will happen again. Exhibit 10.3 offers an exercise to help you practice savoring good moments.

Let's return to the aroma of that coffee and the delicious smell of fresh baked cookies. As we stay with these wonderful smells and enjoy what they do for us, we are actually enhancing our positive feelings by savoring the experience. We can learn to do this more often and in doing so, increase our sense of well-being.

Find Meaning Through Action and Connection

In Chapter 8, we discussed the grief associated with necessary, living losses for parents when their young adult has a mental health disorder. We noted that the work of grieving often involves acknowledging and accepting your feelings no matter what these may be (sadness, anger, guilt, etc.). Essentially, this means that you stop judging yourself for what you feel. In Chapter 9, we also discussed the importance of developing self-compassion and recommended that parents pay particular attention to their self- or other-blaming thoughts. This focus on feelings and thoughts has been a recurrent theme throughout the book. Here, we shift our focus from feelings and thoughts, which are often private and often deeply internalized,

EXHIBIT 10.3. Savoring Good Moments Exercise

- Check your smartphone for photos of yourself that capture happy moments for you.
- Select two and write down what was happening in your photos.
- When you are finished, savor the moment for 2 minutes.

Note. Data from Hoepper et al. (2019).

to your actions. We encourage you to consider finding meaning and healing through action.

Humans are relational beings; when we do good things for others, our potential to flourish as human beings increases (Nelson et al., 2016). For some parents, getting involved in community service is a way to feel like they are making a difference. Likewise, when we help others, we tend to function much better ourselves.

Now, let's think about some important questions to ask yourself before you proceed. First, how much time and energy do I have to commit to this task I am considering? What do I want to get out of this experience? What skill set do I bring to the table? What are my self-care needs, and how do I plan to meet them? What might I anticipate as potential roadblocks to doing this work, and how can I manage them while attending to my own well-being?

Community Service

Once you have asked and answered the preceding questions, you can begin to explore the various volunteer opportunities within your community. See Exhibit 10.4 for a list of possible community volunteer options and online resources to aid in your exploration. It's important to keep in mind the process of finding the "best fit" volunteer experience may take some time. You might need to try more than one option before finding the one that is right for you.

Mental Health Advocacy

Parents can also find a sense of purpose by taking on the very issues their young adults are facing through engaging in mental health advocacy. In his work, Feiler (2020) talks about the merit of finding meaning in a "lifequake" experience by searching and advocating (or promoting) for a cause greater than ourselves. This can be

> **EXHIBIT 10.4. Community Volunteer Possibilities and Online Resources**
>
> In-person opportunities:
> - Prepare/serve food (e.g., local food pantry; prepare and deliver for Meals-on-Wheels program)
> - Build homes (e.g., Habitat for Humanity)
> - Mentor youth (e.g., Big Brothers, Big Sisters, Head Start, coach a youth sports team; after-school programs)
> - Support seniors (e.g., be a companion, transport seniors, aid in household chores)
> - Shelter animals (e.g., rescue animals, foster animals)
> - Conserve the environment (e.g., participate in environmental clean-ups)
>
> Online resources:
> - VolunteerMatch: https://www.volunteermatch.org
> - JustServe: https://www.JustServe.org
> - Engage: https://www.engage.pointsoflight.org

tremendously gratifying and fulfilling work for parents; however, we offer a caveat here. For many parents, the experiences associated with being a mental health advocate can be associated with all kinds of feelings, ranging from frustration and anger to devastation. It can feel demoralizing to put time and effort toward such a cause and have little to show for it at times. Such work can lead you to revisit and reexperience what you have been through or continue to go through with your own adult child. We say this not to dissuade you but rather to prepare you to enter this experience with your eyes wide open.

Mental health advocacy can involve a range of activities aimed at making positive change in mental health care, however small, for others (Friedman-Wheeler & Bodenlos, 2023).

For example, the desire to improve access and quality of treatment for all young adults and others who experience mental health disorders can take many forms. Table 10.1 contains examples of both direct and indirect forms of mental health advocacy. The constructive channeling of these emotions and the practice of fierce compassion for others can empower parents and other family members.

Both courses of action, community service and mental health advocacy, can be powerful sources of healing for parents. Remember, with either option, these efforts can often exact an emotional toll on parents. For example, if their contributions are overlooked, devalued, or do not appear to make a significant impact, parents may become disillusioned. It is important to keep in mind that there is value in the effort itself, regardless of the outcome. We underscore the importance of having realistic expectations, and knowing things can happen that are out of your control.

Regardless of the actions you take, advocacy or community service, it is crucial that you practice self-care and self-compassion as you work toward your goals. Please remember what we've talked with you about, baby steps, "taking in the good," breathing, and working to remain in the present as vital tools for your journey.

COMING FULL CIRCLE

We began this book with the assertion that emerging adults today face unprecedented challenges as they move toward full-fledged adulthood. They are a diverse population that cannot be easily categorized. Generally speaking, we noted that some young adults at one end of the continuum appear to be flourishing and launching successfully into full-fledged adulthood, while others, at the opposite end of the continuum, are struggling to get off the ground because their psychological distress is severe.

TABLE 10.1. Examples of Mental Health Advocacy

Type of advocacy	Examples
Direct advocacy	• Attend to your choice of words and encourage others to use affirmative language (e.g., "person living with bipolar illness") that preserves the dignity of all persons who are in psychological distress and/or diagnosed with mental health disorders. • Consider sharing your personal experiences with mental health issues and the mental health system. • Actively encourage others to seek therapy when they are in psychological distress. • Volunteer for a crisis helpline (e.g., National Suicide Prevention Lifeline) or other social services agency.
Indirect advocacy	• Lobby for increased funding and improved mental health services by speaking with legislators and public policymakers at the local, state, and/or national levels. • Engage in fundraising efforts (e.g., organized walk or run) for mental health organizations and donate to community-based mental health agencies and organizations (e.g., local affiliates of the NAMI or MHA). • Help organize or participate in MHA-sponsored mental health screenings or educational program events. • Educate others about the importance of mental health and treatment through blogging, podcasting, and/or other social media. • Create a product that brings attention to mental health and donate a portion of the proceeds to a mental health agency or organization.

Note. MHA = Mental Health America; NAMI = National Alliance on Mental Illness.

Parents likewise are on a continuum in terms of what the situation with their young adult demands of them. For some, there are relatively few demands placed on them. For another set of parents, the demands come and go. Still others may be on stand-by status almost 24/7 as their adult child struggles. Parents need to work on the skills related to various pivot points, stay emotionally regulated and centered, and focus on their own self-care, regardless of the status of their young adult. For most parents, this involves entering a new normal where the terrain is often rocky and unfamiliar.

Let's return to the stories of our families and apply the continuum model to their unique situations as we understand how these parents are managing their new normal.

Anne's Parents

Anne's mother, Claire, related the following update:

> It is one day at a time with Anne. She was doing really well for a while . . . we got her into a partial hospitalization program after her diagnosis. The staff there did a great job teaching her about bipolar disorder, all about meds, the importance of maintaining a routine, getting consistent sleep and a healthy lifestyle. Anne still plans on going back to school again and completing her undergraduate degree.
>
> She started taking a yoga class and she was maintaining a daily mood log as part of her cognitively based therapy. She got a job working as an assistant at the wildlife refuge near our town. Everything was going great . . . but then she stopped taking her meds again without telling us. Thankfully her boss was understanding because she has a brother who was diagnosed with bipolar disorder.
>
> It feels to me like one step forward and one step back sometimes. I still worry and have many sleepless nights. I try hard to think more positively about Anne's future. But it is

really a struggle . . . it's like a constant looming fear—it never seems to go away. The thought that my child's life is not the same as everyone else's. . . . And yet, I have hope. Her medication is working now. I embrace the good days. Even though I know there are going to be bad days. I am living much more in the present and choosing to focus on what's going well. When I was a little girl, I played the piano. So I bought myself a keyboard recently just for me and I feel good when I play.

Anne's father, Stan, approaches the situation in a different way:

Hey, there is medication, and it seems to be working. I know the social worker said there is a danger of discontinuing meds with a lot of people who have bipolar disorder. Now I understand a little more why Claire has seemed so out of control with all this because of her grandfather's mental illness. But for now, Anne's doing pretty well. So my feeling is, if it ain't broke, don't fix it. I wish Claire would feel the same way. Honestly, I get really uncomfortable when she gets so worked up.

For Stan his pragmatic approach seems to work for him. Stan, unlike many parents, does not appear to be bothered by the stigma associated with mental illness. However, his tendency to push away strong emotions, perhaps even his own, creates added tension in his partnership with Claire.

On the other hand, Claire has a family history of keeping mental illness a secret. For her, it is one day at a time. She takes the good days with the bad days while making an intentional decision to focus on what is going well. Each parent is finding a way to cope with what has happened in their family.

Parents of young adults in severe psychological distress and those with specific mental health disorders are often on guard all the time. They feel on edge constantly and forget to look for the small positive signs along the way. Anne has been diagnosed with an illness that will likely be with her for the rest of her adult life. The medication and therapy are helping her for now; however, at any time, she could make the decision to stop taking the medication or discontinue therapy—or both. If Anne were to discontinue treatment, Stan and Claire may feel like they were back at square one.

Daniel's Parents

Daniel's mother, Lucia, said the following:

> Daniel is doing better. He is enrolled at the community college and has one last semester before he earns his associate degree. He is studying computers and has a job working in the computer lab at school. The staff there really like him. Daniel has a wonderful new girlfriend. They are looking for an apartment together for the fall semester. Arturo doesn't approve of course. I think he still can't seem to get over the fact that Daniel lost his baseball scholarship. I think it was more his wish for Daniel to play for the major leagues than it was Daniel's dream.
>
> Me? I'm better. Things were not so good at home for a time. I am talking with our priest, Father Paul, on a more regular basis. I even dragged Arturo along with me. Father Paul is really trying to help Arturo understand that depression is a brain disorder. He's trying to help us learn how to better communicate with one another. Father Paul also suggested that I consider volunteering. So . . . I've been working at a community Hispanic youth program. I've been tutoring an 8-year-old boy named Sebastian for the past month or so. He was born with fetal alcohol syndrome and is having lots of trouble at school. His home life isn't the best. His mom just got out of a rehab program and has dealt with alcohol abuse for a long time. He is such a sweet kid. It is so rewarding. It has taken my mind off worrying about Daniel.

Lucia's story illustrates more the midpoint along our continuum. She seems to express optimism for Daniel's future. However, this is tempered perhaps by the awareness that Daniel's plans for his life have been substantially altered. His path is still uncertain, and she fears that his depression may recur.

Daniel's father, Arturo, is still not able to fully accept what Daniel is going through.

> I don't mind so much talking with the priest. He gives me information to think about, and I do. But I still don't get why Daniel can't just snap out of this and "be a man." Lucia can go off and do her work with another kid, but I'm still stuck on my son. It just doesn't make sense to me. I still have hopes for him playing Major League baseball at some point. My priest tells me that may not be possible, though. I also hope Daniel will stick with this new girlfriend, and eventually I will have a little grandson to teach to play ball.

Arturo was more receptive to Father Paul's attempts to provide him with information about Daniel's depression and anxiety than he might have been with a stranger, such as a mental health provider. Talking with the priest is a baby step toward understanding the nature of Daniel's depression—that is, why he slept so much and seemed unmotivated for work. Arturo and Lucia's sessions with the priest also focused on how they communicate with each other and what might need to change. One can hope that by learning to communicate more effectively with Lucia, Arturo will also increase his ability to communicate with Daniel. He may be open in the future to examining his interactions with Daniel and what possible messages were sent during his past interactions that may have contributed to his son's depression.

Jessie's Mother

Jessie's mother, Rachel, said the following:

> Jessie is now seeing her therapist online. She was lucky that her old boss at Planet Fitness took her back again and that she had the insurance to cover her telehealth sessions. Because there are no therapists in this area that I don't know, at least on a casual basis, and Jessie was so adamant about not going to anyone that I know, she actually drove nearly an hour and a half to have her initial meeting in person with her therapist. I am really glad she decided to do this. She appears to be learning a lot about herself and seems to be managing her anxiety pretty well.
>
> She has a boyfriend named Luke. He's so good to her. They love to hike the mountain trails and kayak on the lakes around the area. In addition, Jessie has recently switched to a new full-time job at a company that sells organic vitamins. She absolutely loves it. She did so well that the owner of the company offered her a promotion to manager. She is thrilled because it pays well and has great benefits including much better health care. Her copays for her therapy sessions are now more affordable for her.
>
> Me? I finally decided I wanted therapy for myself. So, I've been going every week for the past several months. I am learning a lot. I am realizing that I never fully grieved the loss of my husband. I was so wrapped up in taking care of my kids as a single parent and trying to keep them on an even keel. Yeah, that "supermom" thing really worked against me. I am also learning practical tools like mindfulness meditation and learning to pay more attention to my thoughts and the times when my negative self-talk (a.k.a. my "inner drill sergeant") can increase my anxiety. I am also reconnecting with my love of running and being physically active. For me, physical activity has always been my go-to when I am struggling. And with everything going on with Jessie, I lost track of that.

As things stand at present, Rachel is optimistic about her daughter's future. Jessie appears to be on more solid footing, and her setback seems to have been a temporary one. In addition, the anxiety she struggled with has diminished, allowing her to resume the tasks that are often associated with this stage of emerging adulthood. For Rachel, Jessie's anxiety may have been a catalyst for her own healing. Rachel suggests that her daughter's struggles have kick-started her own commitment to self-growth. Her experience with Jessie triggered feelings of sadness and loss from the death of her spouse. This kind of snowballing effect is not uncommon with such a significant loss.

In her current situation, Rachel is experiencing what we have termed a temporary loss, where her daughter has struggled and appears to be back on track. It is likely that she will continue her journey forward into adulthood. There is a very real possibility that Rachel will be able to pivot to the compeer role with her daughter.

Ian's Father

Ian's father, Pete, said the following:

> I'm proud of Ian. I think he's on a much better track now. I've seen some changes in him since he started his therapy. He seems like he is a lot easier on himself these days and is more self-confident. He finally realized it wasn't the end of the world that it took him a little longer to graduate. Ian's looking for a job now . . . he's decided he's going to take some time off before he goes to graduate school for his MBA. I think this is a great decision, and the fact that he doesn't place that demand on himself is evidence of his growth. He knows he's loved, and he doesn't have to keep on proving himself.

During the following summer break, the two of us hiked part of the Appalachian Trail, from Maine to Pennsylvania. It was one of the best times we've ever had together. I guess, in retrospect, it has been one of the few times that the "no phone" rule wasn't even an issue. No phones or computers, just the most gorgeous mountains you've ever seen. We talked and laughed and enjoyed each other's company. It was the best of times as a parent. Before we each said our goodbyes, we promised each other that within the next 5 years, he and I are going back to finish where we left off and complete the trail.

Me? I'm starting to think about dating again. It has been a long time since I've taken the risk and put myself out there. I figure that I need to practice what I preach and be willing to experience being vulnerable myself. I realized that I may have been afraid I couldn't be a proper dad to Ian and be a partner to someone. Now, I know that there is room enough for me to have both.

Pete's story illustrates what many parents long for—a strong emotional connection with their adult child. The companionship that Pete and his son enjoyed on the Appalachian Trail can be found in many ways and contexts. What is most important is that your relationship with your adult child be characterized by warmth, closeness, respect, and trust. Although Ian still has work ahead of him in terms of finding his place in the world, he appears to be well on his way in his journey to adulthood. However, Peter's words imply that his journey as a parent is not yet over either.

For each of these parents, the prospect of envisioning a future relationship with their adult child is both energizing and a bit intimidating. Although none of us knows what the future holds, we do know there can be a wide range of outcomes when a young adult is struggling with psychological distress. The parents we've described throughout our book have experienced the challenges and losses as well as the joys of life with their emerging adults.

SUMMARY

As we stated earlier in the book, being a parent of a young adult in psychological distress is most assuredly not for the faint of heart. It often leaves the parent feeling broken and in need of repair. Although many of us aspire to one day have a more mutual give-and-take relationship with our adult child, like that embodied in the compeer role, this is not always possible to achieve in a lasting way. For some parents, compeer is a role they pivot into for a time, but then find they must pivot to a different role based on the needs of their young adult. At the same time, balancing their efforts for their adult child with their own self-care will be crucial. As we saw with our parents and their adult children, the road is often long, bumpy, and hard to predict. Nonetheless, each parent was able to focus on their own needs and reconnect or make a new connection to activities that enhanced their own well-being, and, as in the case of Lucia, also contributed to the larger community.

In this chapter, we touched base one last time with our parents and their emerging adults who are at the threshold of adulthood. Stan and Claire, Arturo and Lucia, Rachel, and Peter face the future with a sense of hope while recognizing there will be challenges ahead. By sharing their respective journeys, our main focus has been to offer you information, tools, and techniques to help you stay on track and centered as you contend with the ups and downs of parenting. Perhaps most important, we stressed the need to take care of yourself so you can be available to your young adult when they struggle.

Remember, most times, change happens in small steps rather than giant leaps. Expect to take a step backward on occasion as you continue your journey. The good times (diamonds) and the bad times (stones) ebb and flow throughout life depending on developmental stage and other situational circumstances, like the onset of mental health issues. At this point, your tote bag is full of many useful tools for the road ahead. The important thing for you as a parent of a young adult in psychological distress to do is to *use* the tools. Don't let them collect dust in the corner. You have made it to this point, Mom and Dad. We believe you can do this—and don't forget the belly laughs!

POINTS TO POCKET

- The future for parents of adult children with mental health disorders involves hope and challenge.
- The compeer role is one of equals or peers with mutual respect for each other's choices.
- When an emerging adult is in psychological distress, the pivot to the compeer role may be delayed, but needn't be forgotten.
- Meaning-making after a lifequake can often be found in taking up a cause greater than yourself. This can be done through community service or advocacy.
- There's a Swedish proverb—Add a golden edge to your everyday. Learn to savor the positives in your life.

REFERENCES

Abramson, A. (2022, January 1). Children's mental health is in crisis. *Monitor on Psychology*, *53*(1), 69. https://www.apa.org/monitor/2022/01/special-childrens-mental-health

Abreu, R. L., Sostre, J. P., Gonzalez, K. A., Lockett, G. M., & Matsuno, E. (2022). *"I am afraid for those kids who might find death preferable"*: Parental figures' reactions and coping strategies to bans on gender affirming care for transgender and gender diverse youth. *Psychology of Sexual Orientation and Gender Diversity*, *9*(4), 500–510. https://doi.org/10.1037/sgd0000495

Abreu, R. L., Sostre, J. P., Gonzalez, K. A., Lockett, G. M., Matsuno, E., & Mosley, D. V. (2022). Impact of gender-affirming care bans on transgender and gender diverse youth: Parental figures' perspective. *Journal of Family Psychology*, *36*(5), 643–652. https://doi.org/10.1037/fam0000987

The Academy for Professional Excellence. (2015). *The two wolves: A Cherokee story.* https://www.theacademy.sdsu.edu/wp-content/uploads/2015/06/two-wolves-cherokee-story.pdf

Alderson, C. (2020). *Never let go: How to parent your child through mental illness*. Ebury Digital.

Alpert, J. E., McDonald, W. M., Nemeroff, C. B., & Rodriquez, C. (2022, July). *The use of psychedelic and empathogenic agents for mental health conditions* [Position statement]. American Psychiatric Association. https://www.psychiatry.org/getattachment/d5c13619-ca1f-491f-a7a8-b7141c800904/Position-Use-of-Psychedelic-Empathogenic-Agents.pdf

American College Health Association. (2022). *American College Health Association-National College Health Assessment III: Fall 2021 Reference Group Executive Summary.* https://www.acha.org/wp-content/uploads/2024/07/NCHA-III_FALL_2021_REFERENCE_GROUP_EXECUTIVE_SUMMARY.pdf

American Psychiatric Association. (2000). *Diagnostic and statistical manual of mental disorders* (4th ed., text rev.). https://doi.org/10.1176/appi.books.9780890425787

American Psychiatric Association. (2022). *Diagnostic and statistical manual of mental disorders* (5th ed., text rev.). https://doi.org/10.1176/appi.books.9780890425787

Arnett, J. J. (2000). Emerging adulthood. A theory of development from the late teens through the twenties. *American Psychologist, 55*(5), 469–480. https://doi.org/10.1037/0003-066X.55.5.469

Arnett, J. J. (2007). Emerging adulthood: What is it, and what is it good for? *Child Development Perspectives, 1*(2), 68–73. https://doi.org/10.1111/j.1750-8606.2007.00016.x

Arnett, J. J. (2015). *Emerging adulthood: The winding road from the late teens through the twenties.* Oxford University Press. https://doi.org/10.1093/acprof:oso/9780199929382.001.0001

Arnett, J. J., Žukauskienė, R., & Sugimura, K. (2014). The new life stage of emerging adulthood at ages 18–29 years: Implications for mental health. *The Lancet Psychiatry, 1*(7), 569–576. https://doi.org/10.1016/S2215-0366(14)00080-7

Baker, F. A., Metcalf, O., Varker, T., & O'Donnell, M. (2018). A systematic review of the efficacy of creative arts therapies in the treatment of adults with PTSD. *Psychological Trauma: Theory, Research, Practice, and Policy, 10*(6), 643–651. https://doi.org/10.1037/tra0000353

Bakhshaie, J., Rogers, A. H., Kauffman, B. Y., Tran, N., Buckner, J. D., Ditre, J. W., & Zvolensky, M. J. (2019). Emotion dysregulation as an explanatory factor in the relation between negative affectivity and non-medical use of opioid in a diverse young adult sample. *Addictive Behaviors, 95*, 103–109. https://doi.org/10.1016/j.addbeh.2019.02.025

Balban, M. Y., Neri, E., Kogon, M. M., Weed, L., Nouriani, B., Jo, B., Holl, G., Zeitzer, J. M., Spiegel, D., & Huberman, A. D. (2023). Brief structured respiration practices enhance mood and reduce physiological arousal. *Cell Reports Medicine*, 4(1), Article 100895. https://doi.org/10.1016/j.xcrm.2022.100895

Baldessarini, R. J., Tondo, L., & Hennen, J. (2003). Treatment-latency and previous episodes: Relationships to pretreatment morbidity and response to maintenance treatment in bipolar I and II disorders. *Bipolar Disorders*, 5(3), 169–179. https://doi.org/10.1034/j.1399-5618.2003.00030.x

Barkham, M., & Lambert, M. J. (2021). The efficacy and effectiveness of psychological therapies. In M. Barkham, W. Lutz, & L. G. Castonguay (Eds.), *Bergin and Garfield's handbook of psychotherapy and behavior change* (pp. 135–189). John Wiley & Sons.

Bennett, N., & Lemoine, G. J. (2014, January–February). What VUCA really means for you. *Harvard Business Review*. https://hbr.org/2014/01/what-vuca-really-means-for-you

Boyes, A. (2013, January 17). *50 common cognitive distortions*. https://www.psychologytoday.com/us/blog/in-practice/201301/50-common-cognitive-distortions

Bradley-Geist, J. C., & Olson-Buchanan, J. B. (2014). Helicopter parents: An examination of the correlates of over-parenting of college students. *Education + Training*, 56(4), 314–328. https://doi.org/10.1108/ET-10-2012-0096

Bryant, F. B., & Smith, J. L. (2015). Appreciating life in the midst of adversity: Savoring in relation to mindfulness, reappraisal, and meaning. *Psychological Inquiry*, 26(4), 315–321. https://doi.org/10.1080/1047840X.2015.1075351

Bryant, F. B., & Veroff, J. (2007). *Savoring: A new model of positive experience*. Lawrence Erlbaum Associates.

Center for Collegiate Mental Health. (2022, January). *2021 annual report*. https://ccmh.psu.edu/assets/docs/2021-CCMH-Annual-Report.pdf

Center for Prolonged Grief. (n.d.). [Home page]. Columbia University School of Social Work. https://prolongedgrief.columbia.edu

Centers for Disease Control and Prevention. (2016). *Sexually transmitted disease surveillance 2015*. U.S. Department of Health and Human Services. https://www.cdc.gov/std/stats/archive/STD-Surveillance-2015-print.pdf

Centers for Disease Control and Prevention. (2020). *Facts about suicide*. https://www.cdc.gov/suicide/facts/index.html

Chang, C. H. C., Nastase, S. A., Zadbood, A., & Hasson, U. (2024). How a speaker herds the audience: Multi-brain neural convergence over time during naturalistic storytelling. *Social Cognitive and Affective Neuroscience, 19*(1), nsae059. https://doi.org/10.1093/scan/nsae059

Clay, R. L. (2024). Policy makers are taking aim at women & LGBTQ+ individuals. *The Monitor, 55*(1), 52. https://www.apa.org/monitor/2024/01/trends-policy-developments-women-lgbtq

Close, G. (2010, March 18). *Mental illness: The stigma of silence.* HuffPost. https://www.huffpost.com/entry/mental-illness-the-stigma_b_328591

Collins, L. (2017). *Unfiltered: No shame, no regrets, just me.* Harper.

Craig, C., Hiskey, S., & Spector, A. (2020). Compassion focused therapy: A systematic review of its effectiveness and acceptability in clinical populations. *Expert Review of Neurotherapeutics.* https://doi.org/10.1080/14737175.2020.1746184

Croucher, S. M., Nguyen, T., & Rahmani, D. (2020). Prejudice toward Asian-Americans in the Covid-19 pandemic: The effects of social media use in the United States. *Frontiers in Communication, 5*(39), 1–12. https://doi.org/10.3389/fcomm.2020.00039

Deleuze, J., Maurage, P., Schimmenti, A., Nuyens, F., Melzer, A., & Billieux, J. (2019). Escaping reality through videogames is linked to an implicit preference for virtual over real-life stimuli. *Journal of Affective Disorders, 245*, 1024–1031. https://doi.org/10.1016/j.jad.2018.11.078

Deloitte. (2016, June). *Deloitte Global Mobile Consumer Survey 2016: U.S. edition.* https://www2.deloitte.com/content/dam/Deloitte/us/Documents/technology-media-telecommunications/us-global-mobile-consumer-survey-2016-executive-summary.pdf

Denver, J. (1981). Some days are diamonds [Song]. On *Some days are diamonds.* RCA Records.

De Rozario, M. R., Van Velzen, L. S., Davies, P., Rice, S. M., Davey, C. G., Robinson, J., Alvarez-Jimenez, M., Allott, K., McKechnie, B., Felmingham, K. L., & Schmaal, L. (2021). Mental images of suicide: Theoretical framework and preliminary findings in depressed youth attending outpatient care. *Journal of Affective Disorders, 4*, Article 100114. https://doi.org/10.1016/j.jadr.2021.100114

de Sousa Fernandes, M. S., Ordônio, T. F., Santos, G. C. J., Santos, L. E. R., Calazans, C. T., Gomes, D. A., & Santos, T. M. (2020). Effects of physical exercise on neuroplasticity and brain function: A systematic review in human and animal studies. *Neural Plasticity*, *2020*, Article 8856621. https://doi.org/10.1155/2020/8856621

Doka, K. J. (1989). Disenfranchised grief. In K. J. Doka (Ed.), *Disenfranchised grief: Recognizing hidden sorrow* (pp. 3–12). Lexington Books/ D. C. Heath and Company.

Douglas, A. (2023, May 26). Personal perspective: What I've figured out about being a parent of a young adult. *Psychology Today*. https:// www.psychologytoday.com/us/blog/midlife-reimagined/202305/ midlife-parenting

Drazdowski, T. K. (2016). A systematic review of the motivations for the non-medical use of prescription drugs in young adults. *Drug and Alcohol Dependence*, *162*, 3–25. https://doi.org/10.1016/j.drugalcdep. 2016.01.011

Dunn, J. (2023, April 7). When someone is upset, ask this one question. *The New York Times*. https://www.nytimes.com/2023/04/07/well/ emotions-support-relationships.html

Eisenberg, N., Cumberland, A., & Spinrad, T. L. (1998). Parental socialization of emotion. *Psychological Inquiry*, *9*(4), 241–273. https://doi.org/ 10.1207/s15327965pli0904_1

Fables of Aesop. (n.d.). *The tree and the reed*. https://fablesofaesop.com/ the-tree-and-the-reed.html

Feiler, B. (2020). *Life is in the transitions: Mastering change at any age*. Penguin Press.

Flückiger, C., Del Re, A. C., Wampold, B. E., & Horvath, A. O. (2018). The alliance in adult psychotherapy: A meta-analytic synthesis. *Psychotherapy*, *55*(4), 316–340. https://doi.org/10.1037/pst0000172

Fredrickson, B. L. (1998). What good are positive emotions? *Review of General Psychology*, *2*(3), 300–319. https://doi.org/10.1037/1089-2680.2.3.300

Fredrickson, B. L. (2013). Positive emotions broaden and build. In P. Devine & A. Plant (Eds.), *Advances in experimental social psychology* (Vol. 47, pp. 1–53). Academic Press. https://doi.org/10.1016/B978-0-12-407236-7.00001-2

Friedman-Wheeler, D. G., & Bodenlos, J. S. (2023). *Being the change: A guide for advocates and activists on staying healthy, inspired, and driven*. American Psychological Association. https://doi.org/10.1037/ 0000330-000

Gitterman, A., & Knight, C. (2019). Non-death loss: Grieving for the loss of familiar place and for precious time and associated opportunities. *Clinical Social Work Journal, 47*(2), 147–155. https://doi.org/10.1007/s10615-018-0682-5

Glasser, A., Abudayyeh, H., Cantrell, J., & Niaura, R. (2019). Patterns of e-cigarette use among youth and young adults: Review of the impact of e-cigarettes on cigarette smoking. *Nicotine and Tobacco Research, 21*(10), 1320–1330. https://doi.org/10.1093/ntr/nty103

Goleman, D. (2005). *Emotional intelligence: Why it can matter more than IQ*. Random House.

Gonidakis, F., Lemonoudi, M., Charila, D., & Varsou, E. (2018). A study on the interplay between emerging adulthood and eating disorder symptomatology in young adults. *Eating and Weight Disorders, 23*(6), 797–805. https://doi.org/10.1007/s40519-018-0552-8

Goodwin, R. D., Dierker, L. C., Wu, M., Galea, S., Hoven, C. W., & Weinberger, A. H. (2022). Trends in U.S. depression prevalence from 2015 to 2020: The widening treatment gap. *American Journal of Preventive Medicine, 63*(5), 726–733. https://doi.org/10.1016/j.amepre.2022.05.014

Goodwin, R. D., Weinberger, A. H., Kim, J. H., Wu, M., & Galea, S. (2020). Trends in anxiety among adults in the United States, 2008–2018: Rapid increases among young adults. *Journal of Psychiatric Research, 130*, 441–446. https://doi.org/10.1016/j.jpsychires.2020.08.014

Gorman, K. S., Bruns, C., Chin, C., Fitzpatrick, N., Koenig, L., LeViness, P., & Sokolowski, K. (2020). *Association for University and College Counseling Center Directors Annual Survey*. https://www.aucccd.org/assets/documents/Survey/2019-2020%20Annual%20Report%20FINAL%20March-2021.pdf

Gottman, J. (1998). *Raising an emotionally intelligent child: The heart of parenting*. Simon & Schuster.

Gottman, J. M., Katz, L. F., & Hooven, C. (1996). Parental meta-emotion philosophy and the emotional life of families: Theoretical models and preliminary data. *Journal of Family Psychology, 10*(3), 243. https://doi.org/10.1037/0893-3200.10.3.243

Graupensperger, S., Fleming, C. B., Jaffe, A. E., Rhew, I. C., Patrick, M. E., & Lee, C. M. (2021). Changes in young adults' alcohol and marijuana use, norms, and motives from before to during the COVID-19 pandemic.

The Journal of Adolescent Health, 68(4), 658–665. https://doi.org/10.1016/j.jadohealth.2021.01.008

Gregg, L., Haddock, G., Emsley, R., & Barrowclough, C. (2014). Reasons for substance use and their relationship to subclinical psychotic and affective symptoms, coping, and substance use in a nonclinical sample. *Psychology of Addictive Behaviors*, 28(1), 247–256. https://doi.org/10.1037/a0034761

Guare, R., Guare, C., & Dawson, P. (2019). *Smart but scattered—and stalled: 10 steps to help young adults use their executive skills to set goals, make a plan, and successfully leave the nest.* Guilford Press.

Guarino, H., Mateu-Gelabert, P., Teubl, J., & Goodbody, E. (2018). Young adults' opioid use trajectories: From nonmedical prescription opioid use to heroin, drug injection, drug treatment and overdose. *Addictive Behaviors*, 86, 118–123. https://doi.org/10.1016/j.addbeh.2018.04.017

Gupta, P. S., & Kalagher, K. M. (2021). Where there is (no) smoke, there is still fire: A review of trends, reasons for use, references and harm perceptions of adolescent and young adult electronic cigarette use. *Current Pediatrics Reports*, 9(3), 47–51. https://doi.org/10.1007/s40124-021-00240-1

Hahm, H. C., Xavier Hall, C. D., Garcia, K. T., Cavallino, A., Ha, Y., Cozier, Y. C., & Liu, C. (2021). Experiences of COVID-19-related anti-Asian discrimination and affective reactions in a multiple race sample of U.S. young adults. *BMC Public Health*, 21(1), Article 1563. https://doi.org/10.1186/s12889-021-11559-1

Hanson, M. (2022). *College enrollment & student demographic statistics.* Education Data Initiative. https://educationdata.org/college-enrollment-statistics

Hanson, R. (2010). *Taking in the good: Do positive experiences stick to your ribs?* https://www.psychologytoday.com/intl/blog/your-wise-brain/201002/taking-in-the-good

Hanson, R. (2013). *Hardwiring happiness: The brain science of contentment, calm, and confidence.* Harmony.

Hanson, R., & Mendius, R. (2009). *Buddha's brain: The practical neuroscience of happiness, love & wisdom.* New Harbinger Publications.

Harris, R. (2009). *ACT made simple.* New Harbinger Publications.

Havighurst, S. S., Radovini, A., Hao, B., & Kehoe, C. E. (2020). Emotion-focused parenting interventions for prevention and treatment of child and adolescent mental health problems: A review of the literature. *Current Opinion in Psychiatry, 33*(6), 586–601. https://doi.org/10.1097/YCO.0000000000000647

Hayes, S. C. (2005). *Get out of your mind and into your life.* New Harbinger Publications.

Hemingway, E. (1929). *A farewell to arms.* Gusset & Dunlap.

Hoepper, B. B., Schick, M. R., Carlton, H., & Hoeppner, S. S. (2019). Do self-administered positive psychology exercises work in persons in recovery for problematic substance use? An online randomized survey. *Journal of Substance Abuse Treatment, 99,* 429–431. https://doi.org/10.1016/j.jsat.2019.01.006

Holt, L. J., Ginley, M. K., Pingeon, C., & Feinn, R. (2024). Primed for positive perceptions? Applying the acquired preparedness model to explain college students' e-cigarette use and dependence. *Journal of American College Health, 72*(6), 1734–1744. https://doi.org/10.1080/07448481.2022.2089846

Hughes, A., Williams, M. R., Lipari, R. N., Bose, J., Copello, E. A. P., & Kroutil, L. A. (2016). Prescription drug use and misuse in the United States: Results from the 2015 national survey on drug use and health. *NSDUH Data Review.* https://www.samhsa.gov/data/sites/default/files/NSDUH-FFR2-2015/NSDUH-FFR2-2015.htm

Hwang, H. S. (2019). Why social comparison on Instagram matters: Its impact on depression. *KSII Transactions on Internet and Information Systems, 13*(3), 1626–1638. https://doi.org/10.3837/tiis.2019.03.029

Ilakkuvan, V., Johnson, A., Villanti, A. C., Evans, W. D., & Turner, M. (2019). Patterns of social media use and their relationship to health risks among young adults. *Journal of Adolescent Health, 64*(2), 158–164. https://doi.org/10.1016/j.jadohealth.2018.06.025

Insel, T. (2022). *Healing: Our path from mental illness to mental health.* Penguin Press.

Jaffe, A. E., Blayney, J. A., Graupensperger, S., Stappenbeck, C. A., Bedard-Gilligan, M., & Larimer, M. (2023). Personalized normative feedback for hazardous drinking among college women: Differential outcomes by history of incapacitated rape. *Psychology of Addictive Behaviors, 37*(7), 863–874. https://doi.org/10.1037/adb0000657

Janoff-Bulman, R. (1989). Assumptive worlds and the stress of traumatic events: Applications of the schema construct. *Social Cognition, 7*(2), 113–136. https://doi.org/10.1521/soco.1989.7.2.113

Jordan, A. H., & Litz, B. T. (2014). Prolonged grief disorder: Diagnostic, assessment, and treatment considerations. *Professional Psychology: Research and Practice, 45*(3), 180–187. https://doi.org/10.1037/a0036836

Jordan, C. J., & Andersen, S. L. (2017). Sensitive periods of substance abuse: Early risk for the transition to dependence. *Developmental Cognitive Neuroscience, 25,* 29–44. https://doi.org/10.1016/j.dcn.2016.10.004

Kauffman, J. (2002). Introduction. In J. Kauffman (Ed.), *Loss of the assumptive world: A theory of traumatic loss* (pp. 1–12). Brunner-Routledge.

Keeter, S. (2021, March 16). *Many Americans continue to experience mental health difficulties as pandemic enters second year.* Pew Research Center. https://www.pewresearch.org/fact-tank/2021/03/16/many-americans-continue-to-experience-mental-health-difficulties-as-pandemic-enters-second-year/

Kennedy, B. (2022). *Good inside: A guide to becoming the parent you want to be.* Harper Wave.

Keramatian, K., Pinto, J. V., Schaffer, A., Sharma, V., Beaulieu, S., Parikh, S. V., & Yatham, L. N. (2022). Clinical and demographic factors associated with delayed diagnosis of bipolar disorder: Data from Health Outcomes and Patient Evaluations in Bipolar Disorder (HOPE-BD) study. *Journal of Affective Disorders, 296,* 506–513. https://doi.org/10.1016/j.jad.2021.09.094

Kessler, D. (2019). *Finding meaning: The sixth stage of grief.* Scribner.

Kessler, R. C., Andrews, G., Colpe, L. J., Hiripi, E., Mroczek, D. K., Normand, S. L. T., Walters, E. E., & Zaslavsky, A. M. (2002). Short screening scales to monitor population prevalences and trends in non-specific psychological distress. *Psychological Medicine, 32*(6), 959–976. https://doi.org/10.1017/S0033291702006074

Kessler, R. C., Berglund, P., Demler, O., Jin, R., Merikangas, K. R., & Walters, E. E. (2005). Lifetime prevalence and age-of-onset distributions of *DSM-IV* disorders in the National Comorbidity Survey Replication. *Archives of General Psychiatry, 62*(6), 593–602. https://doi.org/10.1001/archpsyc.62.6.593

Kessler, R. C., Petukhova, M., Sampson, N. A., Zaslavsky, A. M., & Wittchen, H. U. (2012). Twelve-month and lifetime prevalence and lifetime morbid risk of anxiety and mood disorders in the United States. *International Journal of Methods in Psychiatric Research, 21*(3), 169–184. https://doi.org/10.1002/mpr.1359

Keum, B. T., & Choi, A. Y. (2022). COVID-19 racism, depressive symptoms, drinking to cope motives, and alcohol use severity among Asian American emerging adults. *Emerging Adulthood, 10*(6), 1591–1601. https://doi.org/10.1177/21676968221117421

Kinouani, S., Leflot, C., Vanderkam, P., Auriacombe, M., Langlois, E., & Tzourio, C. (2020). Motivations for using electronic cigarettes in young adults: A systematic review. *Substance Abuse, 41*(3), 315–322. https://doi.org/10.1080/08897077.2019.1671937

Kirkbride, J. B., Anglin, D. M., Colman, I., Dykxhoorn, J., Jones, P. B., Patalay, P., Pitman, A., Soneson, E., Steare, T., Wright, T., & Griffiths, S. L. (2024). The social determinants of mental health and disorder: Evidence, prevention and recommendations. *World Psychiatry, 23*(1), 58–90. https://doi.org/10.1002/wps.21160

Konstam, V. (2013). *Parenting your emerging adult: Launching kids from 18 to 29.* New Horizon Press.

Korb, A. (2015). *The upward spiral: Using neuroscience to reverse the course of depression, one small change at a time.* New Harbinger Publications, Inc.

Koss, M. P., Swartout, K. M., Lopez, E. C., Lamade, R. V., Anderson, E. J., Brennan, C. L., & Prentky, R. A. (2022). The scope of rape victimization and perpetration among national samples of college students across 30 years. *Journal of Interpersonal Violence, 37*(1–2), NP25–NP47. https://doi.org/10.1177/08862605211050103

Kouros, C. D., Pruitt, M. M., Ekas, N. V., Kiriaki, R., & Sunderland, M. (2017). Helicopter parenting, autonomy support, and college students' mental health and well-being: The moderating role of sex and ethnicity. *Journal of Child and Family Studies, 26*(3), 939–949. https://doi.org/10.1007/s10826-016-0614-3

Krieger, H., Young, C. M., Anthenien, A. M., & Neighbors, C. (2018). The epidemiology of binge drinking among college-age individuals in the United States. *Alcohol Research: Current Reviews, 39*(1), 23–30.

Kubler-Ross, E. (2014). *On death and dying: What the dying have to teach doctors, nurses, clergy and their own families* (Reissue ed.). Scribner.

Kujawa, A., Green, H., Compas, B. E., Dickey, L., & Pegg, S. (2020). Exposure to COVID-19 pandemic stress: Associations with depression and anxiety in emerging adults in the United States. *Depression and Anxiety, 37*(12), 1280–1288. https://doi.org/10.1002/da.23109

Kwong, A. S. F., López-López, J. A., Hammerton, G., Manley, D., Timpson, N. J., Leckie, G., & Pearson, R. M. (2019). Genetic and environmental risk factors associated with trajectories of depression symptoms from adolescence to young adulthood. *JAMA Network Open, 2*(6), Article e196587. https://doi.org/10.1001/jamanetworkopen.2019.6587

LaFreniere, L. S. (2023). A primer for training savoring skills in psychotherapy (Part 1): Foundational concepts. *The Evidence Based Practitioner.* Philadelphia Behavior Therapy Association. https://philabta.org/EBP/13245504

Lakshmin, P. (2023). *Real self-care.* Penguin Life.

Lawrence, H. R., Nesi, J., & Schwartz-Mette, R. A. (2022). Suicidal mental imagery: Investigating a novel marker of suicide risk. *Emerging Adulthood, 10*(5), 1216–1221. https://doi.org/10.1177/21676968211001593

Leatherman, S. P. (2003). *Dr. Beach's survival guide.* Yale University Press.

Leiner, M., De la Vega, I., & Johansson, B. (2018). Deadly mass shootings, mental health, and policies and regulations: What we are obligated to do! *Frontiers in Pediatrics, 6*(99), Article 99. https://doi.org/10.3389/fped.2018.00099

Levine, S. L., Holding, A. C., Milyavskaya, M., Powers, T. A., & Koestner, R. (2021). Collaborative autonomy: The dynamic relations between personal goal autonomy and perceived autonomy support in emerging adulthood results in positive affect and goal progress. *Motivation Science, 7*(2), 145–152. https://doi.org/10.1037/mot0000209

Lewsley, J., & Slater, R. (2020, July 28). The effects of racism on physical and mental health. *Medical News Today.* https://www.medicalnewstoday.com/articles/effects-of-racism

Li, W., O'Brien, J. E., Snyder, S. M., & Howard, M. O. (2015). Characteristics of internet addiction/pathological internet use in U.S. university students: A qualitative-method investigation. *PLoS One, 10*(2), Article e0117372. https://doi.org/10.1371/journal.pone.0117372

Linehan, M. M. (1993). *Cognitive-behavioral treatment of borderline personality disorder.* Guilford Press.

Linehan, M. M. (2020). *Building a life worth living.* Random House.

Lipson, S. K., Zhou, S., Abelson, S., Heinze, J., Jirsa, M., Morigney, J., Patterson, A., Singh, M., & Eisenberg, D. (2022). Trends in college student mental health and help-seeking by race/ethnicity: Findings from the National Healthy Minds Study, 2013–2021. *Journal of Affective Disorders, 306,* 138–147. https://doi.org/10.1016/j.jad.2022.03.038

Liu, B. P., Lunde, K. B., Jia, C.-X., & Qin, P. (2020). The short-term rate of non-fatal and fatal repetition of deliberate self-harm: A systematic review and meta-analysis of longitudinal studies. *Journal of Affective Disorders, 273*, 597–603. https://doi.org/10.1016/j.jad.2020.05.072

Liu, R. T., Sheehan, A. E., Walsh, R. F. L., Sanzari, C. M., Cheek, S. M., & Hernandez, E. M. (2019). Prevalence and correlates of non-suicidal self-injury among lesbian, gay, bisexual, and transgender individuals: A systematic review and meta-analysis. *Clinical Psychology Review, 74*, Article 101783. https://doi.org/10.1016/j.cpr.2019.101783

Lowe, K., & Arnett, J. J. (2020). Failure to grow up, failure to pay? Parents' views of conflict over money with their emerging adults. *Journal of Family Issues, 41*(3), 359–382. https://doi.org/10.1177/0192513X19876061

Lythcott-Haims, J. (2021). *Your turn: How to be an adult*. Henry Holt & Co.

MacGregor, P. (1994). Grief: The unrecognized parental response to mental illness in a child. *Social Work, 39*(2), 160–166.

Martin, R. A., & Ford, T. (2018). *The psychology of humor: An integrative approach* (2nd ed.). Academic Press.

McCabe, S. E., Boyd, C. J., Evans-Polce, R. J., McCabe, V. V., Schulenberg, J. E., & Veliz, P. T. (2021). Pills to powder: A 17-year transition from prescription opioids to heroin among US adolescents followed into adulthood. *Journal of Addiction Medicine, 15*(3), 241–244. https://doi.org/10.1097/ADM.0000000000000741

McConville, M. (2020). *Failure to launch: Why your twenty-something hasn't grown and what to do about it*. G. P. Putnam's Sons.

McNulty, K. (2021). *Parenting adult children: A practical guide to navigating your evolving relationship*. Rockridge Press.

Medici, C. R., Videbech, P., Gustafsson, L. N., & Munk-Jørgensen, P. (2015). Mortality and secular trend in the incidence of bipolar disorder. *Journal of Affective Disorders, 183*, 39–44. https://doi.org/10.1016/j.jad.2015.04.032

Mignault, L., Vaillancourt-Morel, M. P., Ramos, B., Brassard, A., & Daspe, M. E. (2022). Is swiping right risky? Dating app use, sexual satisfaction, and risky sexual behavior among adolescents and young adults. *Sexual and Relationship Therapy, 39*(3), 819–842. https://doi.org/10.1080/14681994.2022.2078804

Miller, W. R., & Rollnick, S. (2002). *Motivational interviewing: Preparing people for change* (2nd ed.). Guilford Press.

Miller, W. R., & Rollnick, S. (2012). *Motivational interviewing: Helping people change* (3rd ed.). Guilford Press.

Mitchell, J. (1969). Both sides now [Song]. On *Clouds*. Elektra Records.

Moncrieff, J., Cooper, R. E., Stockmann, T., Amendola, S., Hengartner, M. P., & Horowitz, M. A. (2023). The serotonin theory of depression: A systematic umbrella review of the evidence. *Molecular Psychiatry*, *28*(8), 3243–3256. https://doi.org/10.1038/s41380-022-01661-0

Murawska-Ciałowicz, E., Wiatr, M., Ciałowicz, M., Gomes de Assis, G., Borowicz, W., Rocha-Rodrigues, S., Paprocka-Borowicz, M., & Marques, A. (2021). BDNF impact on biological markers of depression—Role of physical exercise and training. *International Journal of Environmental Research and Public Health*, *18*(14), Article 7553. https://doi.org/10.3390/ijerph18147553

Nasir, L. S., & Lacroix, A. E. (2022). Anxiety and stress in young adults. In P. M. Paulman, R. B. Taylor, A. A. Paulman, & L. S. Nasir (Eds.), *Family medicine: Principles and practice* (pp. 481–488). Springer. https://doi.org/10.1007/978-1-4939-0779-3_136-1

National Center for Health Statistics. (2023). *U.S. Census Bureau, Household Pulse Survey, 2020–2023* [Generated interactively]. https://www.cdc.gov/nchs/covid19/pulse/mental-health.htm

National Institute on Drug Abuse. (2018). *Daily use of marijuana among non-college young adults at all time high*. https://nida.nih.gov/news-events/news-releases/2018/09/daily-use-of-marijuana-among-non-college-young-adults-at-all-time-high

National Institute on Drug Abuse. (2022, August 22). *Marijuana and hallucinogen use among young adults reached all time-high in 2021* [Press release]. https://nida.nih.gov/news-events/news-releases/2022/08/marijuana-and-hallucinogen-use-among-young-adults-reached-all-time-high-in-2021

National Institute on Drug Abuse, & the National Institutes of Health, U.S. Department of Health and Human Services. (2020, September 15). *Vaping & cannabis trends among young adults 19–22* [Press release]. https://nida.nih.gov/research-topics/college-age-young-adults/vaping-cannabis-trends-among-young-adults-infographic

Navarro, T. (2019). *Kintsugi: The Japanese art of embracing the imperfect and loving your flaws*. Sounds True.

Neff, K. (2011). *Self-compassion: The proven power of being kind to yourself.* HarperCollins.

Neff, K. (2021). *Fierce self-compassion: How women can harness kindness to speak up, claim their power, and thrive.* HarperCollins.

Neff, K., & Germer, C. (2018). *The mindful self-compassion workbook.* Guilford Press.

Neimeyer, R. A., Burke, L. A., MacKay, M. M., & van Dyke Stringer, J. G. (2010). Grief therapy and the reconstruction of meaning: From principles to practice. *Journal of Contemporary Psychotherapy, 40*(2), 73–83. https://doi.org/10.1007/s10879-009-9135-3

Nelson, S. K., Layous, K., Cole, S. W., & Lyubomirsky, S. (2016). Do unto others or treat yourself? The effects of prosocial and self-focused behavior on psychological flourishing. *Emotion, 16*(6), 850–861. https://doi.org/10.1037/emo0000178

Nguyen, J. (2022). *Don't believe everything you think.* One Sartori LLC.

Norcross, J. C., & Lambert, M. J. (2018). Psychotherapy relationships that work III. *Psychotherapy, 55*(4), 303–315. https://doi.org/10.1037/pst0000193

Oexle, N., Feigelman, W., & Sheehan, L. (2020). Perceived suicide stigma, secrecy about suicide loss and mental health outcomes. *Death Studies, 44*(4), 248–255. https://doi.org/10.1080/07481187.2018.1539052

Office of the Surgeon General. (2023). *Our epidemic of loneliness and isolation: The U.S. surgeon general's advisory on the healing effects of social connection and community.* U.S. Department of Health and Human Services. https://www.hhs.gov/sites/default/files/surgeon-general-social-connection-advisory.pdf

Olga Phoenix Project. (2013). *Self-care wheel: Healing for social change.* https://olgaphoenix.com/self-care-wheel/

Owczarek, M., Jurek, J., Nolan, E., & Shevlin, M. (2022). Nutrient deficiency profiles and depression: A latent class analysis study of American population. *Journal of Affective Disorders, 317,* 339–346. https://doi.org/10.1016/j.jad.2022.08.100

Parkes, C. (1988). Bereavement as a psychosocial transition: Processes of adaptation to change. *Journal of Social Issues, 44*(3), 53–65. https://doi.org/10.1111/j.1540-4560.1988.tb02076.x

Perrine, S. (2022, September 2). Our kids are in crisis. *AARP Bulletin, 63*(7). https://www.aarp.org/home-family/friends-family/info-2022/teens-mental-health-crisis-causes-warning-signs.html

Peterson, C., & Seligman, M. E. P. (2004). *Character strengths and virtues: A handbook and classification*. Oxford University Press; American Psychological Association.

Pew Research Center. (2024, January 25). *Parents, young adult children and the transition to adulthood*. https://www.pewresearch.org/social-trends/2024/01/25/parents-young-adult-children-and-the-transition-to-adulthood/

Piechaczek, C. E., Pehl, V., Feldmann, L., Haberstroh, S., Allgaier, A. K., Freisleder, F. J., Schulte-Körne, G., & Greimel, E. (2020). Psychosocial stressors and protective factors for major depression in youth: Evidence from a case–control study. *Child and Adolescent Psychiatry and Mental Health, 14*(6). https://doi.org/10.1186/s13034-020-0312-1

Pine, V. R. (1989). Death, loss, and disenfranchised grief. In K. J. Doka (Ed.), *Disenfranchised grief: Recognizing hidden sorrow* (pp. 13–23). Lexington Press.

Pinkowski, J. (2017, December 27). 6 priceless documents that reveal key moments early in Einstein's career. *Mental Floss*. https://www.mentalfloss.com/article/518759/6-priceless-documents-reveal-key-moments-early-einsteins-career

Plett, H. (2015, March 11). *What it means to "hold space" for people, plus eight tips on how to do it well*. https://heatherplett.com/2015/03/hold-space/blog

Plett, H. (2020). *The art of holding space*. Page Two.

Powers, T. A., Koestner, R., & Zuroff, D. C. (2007). Self-criticism, goal motivation, and goal progress. *Journal of Social and Clinical Psychology, 26*(7), 826–840.

Price, C. (2018). *How to break up with your phone*. Ten Speed Press.

Prigerson, H. G., Shear, M. K., & Reynolds, C. F. (2022). Prolonged grief disorder diagnostic criteria—Helping those with maladaptive grief responses. *JAMA Psychiatry, 79*(4), 277–278. https://doi.org/10.1001/jamapsychiatry.2021.4201

Prochaska, J. O., & DiClemente, C. C. (1983). Stages and processes of self-change of smoking: Toward an integrative model of change. *Journal of Consulting and Clinical Psychology, 51*(3), 390–395. https://doi.org/10.1037/0022-006X.51.3.390

Rasmussen, E. E., Punyanunt-Carter, N., LaFreniere, J. R., Norman, M. S., & Kimball, T. G. (2020). The serially mediated relationship between emerging adults' social media use and mental well-being. *Computers in Human Behavior, 102*, 206–213. https://doi.org/10.1016/j.chb. 2019.08.019

Rettner, R. (2010, June 3). Helicopter parents have neurotic kids. *NBC News.* https://www.nbcnews.com/health/health-news/helicopter-parents-have-neurotic-kids-flna1c9446912

Richman-Abdou, K. (2022, March 5). Kintsugi: The centuries-old art of repairing broken pottery with gold. *My Modern Met.* https://mymodernmet.com/kintsugi-kintsukuroi/

Robertson, I., & Cooper, C. L. (2013). Resilience. *Stress and Health, 29*(3), 175–176. https://doi.org/10.1002/smi.2512

Rosenberg, R. B. (2015). *Nonviolent communication. A language of life.* PuddleDancer.

Saakvitne, K. W., & Pearlman, L. A. (1996). *Transforming the pain: A workbook on vicarious traumatization.* W. W. Norton & Company.

Saini, A., Kumar, M., Bhatt, S., Saini, V., & Malik, A. (2020). Cancer causes and treatments. *International Journal of Pharmaceutical Sciences and Research, 11*(7), 3121–3134. https://doi.org/10.13040/IJPSR.0975-8232.11(7).3121-34

Saks, E. R. (2008). *The center will not hold: My journey through madness.* Hachette Books.

Salvatore, P., Tohen, M., Kaur Khalsa, H. M., Baethge, C., Tondo, L., & Baldessarini, R. J. (2007). Longitudinal research on bipolar disorders. *Epidemiologia e Psichiatria Sociale, 16*(2), 109–117. https://doi.org/ 10.1017/S1121189X00004711

Salway, T., Gesink, D., Ferlatte, O., Rich, A. J., Rhodes, A. E., Brennan, D. J., & Gilbert, M. (2021). Age, period, and cohort patterns in the epidemiology of suicide attempts among sexual minorities in the United States and Canada: Detection of a second peak in middle adulthood. *Social Psychiatry and Psychiatric Epidemiology, 56*(2), 283–294. https://doi.org/10.1007/s00127-020-01946-1

Sawyer, A. N., Smith, E. R., & Benotsch, E. G. (2018). Dating application use and sexual risk behavior among young adults. *Sexuality Research & Social Policy: A Journal of the National Sexuality Resource Center, 15*(2), 183–191. https://doi.org/10.1007/s13178-017-0297-6

Sayyah, M. D., Merrick, J. S., Larson, M. D., & Narayan, A. J. (2022). Childhood adversity subtypes and young adulthood mental health problems: Unpacking effects of maltreatment, family dysfunction, and peer victimization. *Children and Youth Services Review, 137,* Article 106455. https://doi.org/10.1016/j.childyouth.2022.106455

Schulenberg, J. E., Johnston, L. D., O'Malley, P. M., Bachman, J. G., Miech, R. A., & Patrick, M. E. (2017). *Monitoring the Future national survey results on drug use, 1975–2016: Vol. II. College students and adults ages 19–55.* Institute for Social Research, The University of Michigan. https://monitoringthefuture.org/wp-content/uploads/2022/08/mtf-vol2_2016.pdf

Schwartz, B. (2004). The tyranny of choice. *Scientific American, 290*(4), 70–75. https://doi.org/10.1038/scientificamerican0404-70

Seligman, M. E. P. (2012). *Flourish: A new understanding of happiness and well-being and how to achieve them.* Atria.

Seligman, M. E. P., Steen, T. A., Park, N., & Peterson, C. (2005). Positive psychology progress: Empirical validation of interventions. *American Psychologist, 60*(5), 410–421. https://doi.org/10.1037/0003-066X.60.5.410

Semahegn, A., Torpey, K., Manu, A., Assefa, N., Tesfaye, G., & Ankomah, A. (2020). Psychotropic medication non-adherence and its associated factors among patients with major psychiatric disorders: A systematic review and meta-analysis. *Systematic Reviews, 9*(1), Article 17. https://doi.org/10.1186/s13643-020-1274-3

Settersten, R. A., Ottusch, T. M., & Schneider, B. (2015). Becoming adult: Meanings of markers to adulthood. In R. Scott & S. Kosslyn (Eds.), *Emerging trends in the social and behavioral sciences* (pp. 1–16). John Wiley & Sons, Inc. https://doi.org/10.1002/9781118900772.etrds0021

Shafir, R. Z. (2003). *The Zen of listening: Mindful communication in the age of distraction.* Quest Books.

Sherlock, M., & Wagstaff, D. L. (2019). Exploring the relationship between frequency of Instagram use, exposure to idealized images, and psychological well-being in women. *Psychology of Popular Media Culture, 8*(4), 482–490. https://doi.org/10.1037/ppm0000182

Singh, B., Olds, T., Curtis, R., Dumuid, D., Virgara, R., Watson, A., Szeto, K., O'Connor, E., Ferguson, T., Eglitis, E., Miatke, A., Simpson, C. E., & Maher, C. (2023). Effectiveness of physical activity interventions for improving depression, anxiety and distress: An overview of systematic reviews. *British Journal of Sports Medicine, 57*(18), 1203–1209. https://doi.org/10.1136/bjsports-2022-106195

Smith, P., & Delgado, H. (2020). Working with non-death losses in counseling: An overview of grief needs and approaches. *Adultspan Journal, 19*(2), 118–127. https://doi.org/10.1002/adsp.12100

Smriti, D., Ambulkar, S., Meng, Q., Kaimal, G., Ramotar, K., Park, S. Y., & Huh-Yoo, J. (2022). Creative arts therapies for the mental health of emerging adults: A systematic review. *The Arts in Psychotherapy, 77*, Article 101861. https://doi.org/10.1016/j.aip.2021.101861

Spitzer, E. G., Crosby, E. S., & Witte, T. K. (2023). Looking through a filtered lens: Negative social comparison on social media and suicidal ideation among young adults. *Psychology of Popular Media, 12*(1), 69–76. https://doi.org/10.1037/ppm0000380

Steinberg, L. (2023). *You and your adult child: How to grow together in challenging times.* Simon & Schuster.

Stephens, G. J., Silbert, L. J., & Hasson, U. (2010). Speaker–listener neural coupling underlies successful communication. *Proceedings of the National Academy of Sciences, 107*(32), 14425–14430. https://doi.org/10.1073/pnas.1008662107

Stoddard, J. A., & Afari, N. (2014). *The big book of ACT metaphors.* New Harbinger Publications.

Stroebe, M., & Schut, H. (1999). The dual process model of coping with bereavement: Rationale and description. *Death Studies, 23*(3), 197–224. https://doi.org/10.1080/074811899201046

Substance Abuse and Mental Health Services Administration. (2017). *Key substance use and mental health indicators in the United States: Results from the 2016 national survey on drug use and health* (HHS publication no. SMA 17–5044, NSDUH series H-52). Center for Behavioral Health Statistics and Quality. https://www.samhsa.gov/data/sites/default/files/cbhsq-reports/NSDUHFFR2017/NSDUHFFR2017.pdf

Substance Abuse and Mental Health Services Administration. (2019). *A practical guide to psychiatric advance directives.* Center for Mental Health Services. https://www.samhsa.gov/resource/ebp/practical-guide-psychiatric-advance-directives

Szuhany, K. L., Malgaroli, M., Miron, C. D., & Simon, N. M. (2021). Prolonged grief disorder: Course, diagnosis, assessment, and treatment. *Focus, 19*(2), 161–172. https://doi.org/10.1176/appi.focus.20200052

Terlizzi, E. P., & Norris, T. (2021). *Mental health treatment among adults: United States, 2020* (Data Brief, No. 419) National Center for Health Statistics. https://doi.org/10.15620/cdc:110593

U.S. Department of Education. (2022, July 29). *Fact sheet: Biden–Harris administration announces two new actions to address youth mental health crisis* [Press release]. https://www.ed.gov/news/press-releases/fact-sheet-biden-harris-administration-announces-two-new-actions-address-youth-mental-health-crisis

Villarroel, M. A., & Terlizzi, E. P. (2020). *Symptoms of depression in young adults: United States, 2019* (NCHS Data Brief. No. 379). U.S. Department of Health and Human Services, Centers for Disease Control and Prevention. https://www.cdc.gov/nchs/products/databriefs/db379.htm

Wakelin, K. D., Perman, G., & Simonds, L. M. (2022). Effectiveness of self-compassion-related interventions for reducing self-criticism: A systematic review and meta-analysis. *Clinical Psychology and Psychotherapy, 29*, 1–25. https://doi.org/10.1002/cpp.2586

Whitlock, J., & Lloyd-Richardson, E. (2019). *Healing self-injury: A compassionate guide for parents and other loved ones.* Oxford University Press.

Williams, D. R. (2018). Stress and the mental health of populations of color: Advancing our understanding of race-related stressors. *Journal of Health and Social Behavior, 59*(4), 466–485. https://doi.org/10.1177/0022146518814251

Willoughby, T., Heffer, T., Good, M., & Magnacca, M. (2021). Is adolescence a time of heightened risk-taking? An overview of types of risk-taking behaviors across age groups. *Developmental Review, 61*, Article 100980. https://doi.org/10.1016/j.dr.2021.100980

Wood, D., Crapnell, T., Lau, L., Bennett, A., Lotstein, D., Ferris, M., & Kuo, A. (2018). Emerging adulthood as a critical stage in the life course. In N. Halfon, C. B. Forrest, R. M. Lerner, & E. M. Faustman (Eds.), *Handbook of life course health development* (pp. 123–143). Springer. https://doi.org/10.1007/978-3-319-47143-3_7

Worden, J. W. (2008). *Grief counseling and grief therapy: A handbook for the mental health practitioner* (4th ed.). Springer. https://doi.org/10.1891/9780826101211

Worden, J. W. (2015). Theoretical perspectives on grief and loss. In J. M. Stillion & T. Attig (Eds.), *Death, dying and bereavement: Contemporary perspectives, institutions & practices* (pp. 91–103). Springer. https://doi.org/10.1891/9780826171429.0007

INDEX

ABOUT THE AUTHORS

Lynne Carroll, PhD, ABPP, is a retired professor of psychology and former director of the graduate program in counseling psychology at the University of North Florida. Throughout her 30+ years in academia, Dr. Carroll taught a myriad of undergraduate and graduate courses in psychology and mental health counseling at universities in Maryland and Pennsylvania. She supervised clinical interns and students' theses and dissertations. Dr. Carroll's research focused on intersecting identities and mental health and has been widely published in peer-reviewed journals and in book chapters. She is the author of a graduate textbook on psychotherapy published in 2010 by Pearson. Dr. Carroll presented papers at numerous national and international conferences. A licensed and board-certified counseling psychologist, her clinical work included the use of evidence-based treatments for anxiety and depression in young adults. She lives in St. Petersburg, Florida with her partner and enjoys painting, boating, and hiking mountain trails in North Carolina.

Paula J. Gilroy, EdD, is a licensed psychologist with over 30 years of clinical experience with young adults. In her practice at a university counseling center, Dr. Gilroy worked with issues ranging from mild anxiety and depression to more serious mental health disorders such as bipolar and posttraumatic stress disorder. As Assistant Director for Training, Dr. Gilroy provided clinical supervision for both master's level students in training and university faculty who were in the process of seeking licensure in Iowa. Dr. Gilroy presented papers at numerous national conferences and coauthored scholarly articles on various topics, with particular interest in mental health clinicians' own experiences with depression and its impact personally and professionally. As the mother of a young adult, Dr. Gilroy has direct experience with the various pivots involved in the parenting process. She lives in Iowa with her husband and their menagerie of three dogs, five cats, and one bunny named Bugz.

Mikal Crawford, EdD, is a licensed psychologist in Maine who has worked with young adults in a university counseling center and in graduate programs in counseling and human relations in Maryland and Maine for over 30 years. In addition to publishing scholarly articles, she presented workshops regionally, nationally, and internationally on self-care issues, rural mental health issues, stress and burnout, and crisis intervention. Dr. Crawford initiated a program on parent adjustment as part of a summer orientation program for parents of young adults heading to college. She worked with parents on learning to pivot from the caretaker role as their young adults enter college. As the mother of two adult daughters, Dr. Crawford understands firsthand many of the challenges and pivots facing parents of young adults. In retirement she enjoys reading, writing, sailing, and traveling with her husband and her therapy dog Riley from their home base in mid-coast Maine.